PATIENTLY INFLUENCED

STEVE STOKL

Patiently Influenced
Copyright © 2019 by Steve Stokl

All rights reserved. No part of this publication may be reproduced, distributed, or transmitted in any form or by any means, including photocopying, recording, or other electronic or mechanical methods, without the prior written permission of the author, except in the case of brief quotations embodied in critical reviews and certain other non-commercial uses permitted by copyright law.

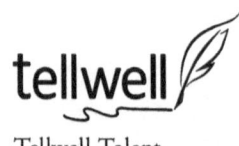

Tellwell Talent
www.tellwell.ca

ISBN
978-0-2288-1730-7 (Hardcover)
978-0-2288-1729-1 (Paperback)
978-0-2288-1731-4 (eBook)

Table of Contents

Introduction 1
Life's Lessons 9
   A Checkup From the Neck Up 11
   A Dance of Intimacy 13
   And We Will Learn 15
   A Lottery Well Spent 16
   An Aged Native Man 17
   An Unknown Hormonal Urge 21
   A Warning Or An Invitation 24
   Believe I'll Find 30
   Dancing to Victory 32
   Everything Matters 35
   False Evidence Appearing Real 37
   Fountain Of Youth 39
   Glass House Living 41
   GUTS 43
   Healing Of Time 45
   Homo Sapien 47
   It's What We Finish 49
   Just Go The Right Way 51
   Life's Marathon Sprint 52
   Live For What You're Here For 53
   Live To Learn To Live 55
   Navigating The Ride 57

    No More 'Yah But' 59
    Numero Uno 61
    Passion Is A Permanent Partner Pact 63
    Recognitionem 65
    Remember The Time 67
    Small Talk 69
    Temperature Temperament 71
    The Protagonist's Antagonist 73
    True Romance 75
    You Can Do It 78
    What If? 80

You and I 83
    A Not So Ugly Ducking 85
    A Slice Of Life 89
    Gregg 92
    Fibro 94
    Insomnia 96
    Mirror Mirror On The Wall 99
    Painfully True 103
    Purgatory Performance 110
    Rise Up and Apologize 112
    Serendipitous Salvation 114
    Soft Place To Fall 117
    That Call In The Night 121

Love 123
    Edified 125
    Give Thanks 127
    I Just Love Her With All My Heart 129
    I'm "Lucky Joe" 131
    Not A Lonely Tale 132
    The Dinner Bell of Love 136
    True Love 143
    Your's 148

Personal 151
   Anne 153
   A Personified Asymptote 160
   A Wick From Keswick 161
   Gotta Feed My Belly 163
   Ironic Age 165
   Lying Supine Is So Divine 166
   Madgie Nation 167
   Mona Lisa 168
   Nulli Secundus 169
   Tapp'n 171
   TGIF 172

Relationships 175
   Alliteration Addiction 177
   Gravitational Relationship Laws 179
   Growing Older and Up 183
   I Should've Known Better 185
   It's All In A Name 186
   Joyful Travailing 189
   Know Where You're Going 190
   Made In The Shade 192
   Marital Manners 194
   No Malice Intended 197
   Our Agenda Doomed Our Dance 200
   Quid Pro Quo 202
   Purple 204
   That First Best Kiss 205
   There Is Only Do 207
   There Is Nothing Quite Like It 209
   Today Is Yesterday 211
   Veni, Vidi, Vici 213
   You Turn The Other Cheek 215
   We Are All Explorers 218

The Big Questions 221
    Choose Your Eternal Thrill 223
    How We Will Dash 229
    It's Showdown 230
    It Takes Time To Understand 232
    This Deal 's Okay 234
    Post Mortem Credo 236
    Remote Control 239
    Truth 241
    What's It Going To Be 244
    Biography 247
    Critical Praise 249

Introduction

My favourite subject during high school was English. I was enthralled with fictional prose: Golding, Leacock, Bronte, and even Shakespeare's tragedies and comedies as well. My teachers, Chuck Calzonetti and Gerry Ward, were instrumental here with their passionate ability to make the characters in the books become alive and so real for me. Poetry on the other hand—Milton, T.S. Elliot, Browning, and others—I found to be a more difficult read. The writers seemed to speak in a unique dialect of English words written in some kind of secret code. Often, despite my best efforts, I simply wasn't able to connect the dots and embrace the full and heartfelt meaningful message that was being delivered. Hence, it was often 'paradise lost' for me.

I never went on to study English at University as I wasn't secure in the belief that I could achieve 90% in these courses. I had decided to become a medical doctor and knew I required good marks to get into medical school. I felt vulnerable, even somewhat insecure, that I'd be able to achieve excellent grades in the subject of English because I believed there was too much subjective dependence on the tutorial assistants or professors own likes/dislikes in grading an English paper. So I veered away from these studies. Instead I studied the natural sciences: the fact based courses of physics, biology, chemistry, mathematics, astronomy (although I did take several philosophy courses), where there would be less subjective opinion influencing my grades by those marking me.

Interestingly, a very recent study by Rey Hernandez-Julian and Christina Peters out of Metropolitan State University of Denver, showed that the better-looking the students are, the greater the difference in grades between online and traditional classes, with the students getting better grades in the classes where they could be seen. Peters said that it wasn't just that more attractive people have other personality traits, or other skills, but it appears to be some type of discrimination on the part of the professors.

This is a 2015 study, the results of which I believe surely would've applied to me in the mid 70's. Heck, if I'd taken English, I probably would've been nailed for sure!

Anyways, after medical school I found myself returning to reading many of the classic books that I hadn't taken time out to read, along with famous pieces of poetry from other countries like India and Japan, besides the very moving and insightful writings of Kalhil Gibran. I then went into Psychiatry which is probably the closest medical discipline allowing me to keep in touch with my original love of English literature.

In 2007 I wrote an award winning book entitled 'Mentally Speaking', published by Volumes. Yet it wasn't a novel of fictional prose that I've always had in mind to write since being a teenager.

I then decided to try and apply myself to writing such a novel. I developed a decent plot along with a half a dozen characters that I wanted to weave into the yarn. Amongst the characters was a pudgy appearing Caucasian man with curly brown hair, a down to earth guy who tended to be discounted and marginalized by many of his peers. Despite this ostracization, he had wonderful street knowledge and virtuous discernment. He would state various affirmations and adages to his peers, and many times he would respond timely with a lyric from a movie or even sing a line from a song to exactly meet the moment, only then to go on quoting the name of the movie or song as if he were footnoting his reference. This was both illuminating, yet annoying to his 'friends', who, for the most part despite his quick wit, summarily regarded him as an imbecile. At any rate as the story progressed he became a very successful song writer and singer and together with the accompaniment of trusted band members and his own electric guitar, he became quite famous. This led me to start to write some songs for this character, and I put together about 15 songs (lyrics without the music).

In the early part of 2014 I entered the International Song Writing Competition out of Nashville, Tennessee and submitted these songs in the 'Lyrics only' category and surprisingly one of them made it into the semi-finals - 'I'm Lucky Joe'.

My middle son Travis belongs to a very promising Indie pop band called The Elwins (who were nominated for a Juno Award in 2016 in 'Breakout Artist of the Year' category) and I showed him and the lead singer Matt Sweeny some of my songs. We had some good laughs around them and at one point my son and I spent a couple of hours together putting a rhythm to one of these songs. It never came to fruition although just this Christmas he took this song (poem) along with a dozen others and stated that for Christmas he was going to write some music for one of these as a gift to me so I am positively anticipating the result of such a loving offer.

In the meanwhile, with all my responsibilities as Chief of Psychiatry and carrying a rather heavy load of complex patients to care for in my private practice, I was realizing that I just wasn't having enough time or energy left over to gather the momentum to sustain the focus necessary to write my fictional story. It also struck me as well that these "songs" that I had been writing were really actually poems, just as all lyrics in music can be viewed.

As such, I decided to modify the songs into poems and, I find myself now (if I may be so bold) being a poet, and I am thoroughly enjoying it. Though if you were to agree with the quote from this year's Oscar nominated movie 'The Big Short' (based upon the Michael Lewis novel, 'The Big Short: Inside the Doomsday Machine), then you'll enjoy poetry as much as you do 'Truth', and most of us live our lives doing all we can to avoid the truth, just ask any Psychiatrist. Now that's just my professional opinion of course. However, being a psychiatrist myself and having shortened an inch over the years to five feet three inches tall, this credentializes me as a true 'shrink'.

Being a psychiatrist is a tremendous trusted privilege to hear and discuss with patients about the intimacy of their suffering, depression, anxiety, relationship challenges, priorities in life, money problems etc. Their overcoming attitude, and ability to persevere and continue to put one foot forward in front of another, despite the trauma, losses, and societal stigmatization they experience, is a daily inspiration to myself as a human being going through my own life's journey. At times their telling of their odyssey (a phrase that they might use) would also strike a chord in me to ponder and often an idea for a song (and now a poem) would germinate. I continue to be fertilized with emotional and thought-provoking issues from my work with my patients which have led to the growth and development of these poems.

For example, I had a woman come in who just happened to regale about a relationship with a fellow that she had been involved with for four months that ended up turning sour and she expressed, "I should have known better, I just should have known better."

I felt that that was an excellent lyric for a song (which I later modified into a poem) only to discover (and then, yes remember) that the Beatles had written a song with that exact title (composed by John Lennon, credited to Lennon-McCartney originally issued on 'A Hard Day's Night' their soundtrack for the film of the same name released July 10 1964).

The fact is, I truly have been "Patiently Influenced" by the individuals who cross the threshold into my office, as together we attempt to understand and alleviate their pain, agony, and hurtful heart by embracing healthier coping strategies to secure a much improved contentment and happiness in their life. It is these individuals, whose confidentiality I have protected with no names nor clue as to who the person is, who have given rise to the lion's share of these poems—my most sincere gratitude to every one of my patients.

In the early fall of 2014 I sent in several poems to Polar Expressions, and quite frankly I was thrilled to learn that they would include one of them - 'There's Nothing Quite Like It', in their November 2014 publication of poetry entitled - The Warbler's Song. Recognition is such a lovely experience.

I want to take this opportunity to very much thank Christine Bacchus who exemplified 'patience personified' by allowing me to revise, revise, revise, wordsmith again and again, alter punctuation etc.; and not once did she complain nor utter a colourful word of displeasure... that I heard!

I am hopeful that these lyrics will be an enjoyable read for anyone who takes the time to peruse these poems. I would guess that if they don't like them at all, then it might be an excellent non-medicinal way of combatting their initial insomnia by reading any of these pages. I believe the reader will also find that there is very little secret code in these poems; the trails to connect the dots are neither arduous nor mysterious. You see, I want the reader to comprehend. No guessing. No disguise. Honest transparency please, and thank you.

To quote a very dear beloved friend of my fathers, Dr. (Professor) Joseph Mileck out of Berkeley University California, who has been acclaimed for his own biographical writings on the late great Herman Hesse, plus himself having written several books of poetry, "... a poem that is not read, is really only half a poem".

Cheers,
Steve Stokl

There are many beautiful women in the world, and some of them too are quite good looking. Borrowing from a line made famous by the Mamas & Papas in 1966 (though written by Lowman Pauling of the "5" Royales and produced by Ralph Bass in 1957), this is dedicated to the One I love.

Psalm 84:1

Consult not your fears but your hopes and your dreams. Think not about your frustrations, but about your unfulfilled potential. Concern yourself not with what you tried and failed in, but with what it is still possible for you to do.

St. John XXIII

Life's Lessons

A Checkup From the Neck Up

Well again I'd been drink'n
and I just wasn't think'n.
I hadn't been eat'n right
and now my pants were too tight.
Seems the city makes you do
what you don't want.
Seems the city makes you become
someone you're not.
I'd rationalized a painful trial
into a permanent disability.
What I'd done to stay young
my grand folk would call silly.
For its a life of heaven
on the road to hell,
and it's the life of hell
taking the road to heaven.
I was bored with beer
always preparing for the next party.
Driving my life's destiny
like a freelance kamikaze.
Tired of offering caresses
to arms that don't embrace.
Empty bowelled of meaning,
having lost what and why I did chase.

For when the feces start fly'n
what will I do?
We don't learn when we win,
only when we lose.
So it's 'bout time I grew a fold
in my frontal lobe,
or the tale to my progeny
will be neither dashing nor bold.

A Dance of Intimacy

A man and a woman
walking hand in hand,
paired hearts pulsating together,
a dance of intimacy
older than time.
The journey is sweet
albeit brief
tasting finer than any wine.

Youth believes in immortality
at least their conduct speaks so.
Ignoring a cemetery's invitation to
remember, what you are, we were,
and what we are, you will be.
True, we'll be a long time
dusty.
Best to take life in big bites.

The world is full of ghosts.
Seems the longer you live
the more haunted you become.
Lessons learned, that
women aren't always right,
however they are never wrong,

and despite the high cost of living,
it is still very popular indeed.

Perpetual forks in the road with
decisions, choices, resolutions
we've willed to make.
Ending up where we are now,
perhaps hurt, lonely, deflated, void,
stricken by shame, guilt, and anger
at ourselves.
Hence immobilized to solve and continue.

Best to know
we've all been there
even better to reach out extending to all.
Realize that if you're always right,
you'll never have anyone left.
That if you want to be a bridge,
you'll have to lie down
and let people walk all over you.

So sleep more than you work
and work more than you party
though certainly party as much as you can.
Go too where you are celebrated
not tolerated.
Be with someone who
makes you laugh.
It's a beautiful denouement.

And We Will Learn

Will something happen to me?
Something special?
Will all I do or not do,
Make sense one day?
Will I truly do something
Meaningful?
Will I have a purpose
In whatever I do?
When we can go anywhere
Pursue any interest
Whether passionately inclined or not
Having no idea of our desire,
We are never lost.
For everything is our teacher
And we will learn.
Most certainly.

A Lottery Well Spent

Who we're born to, and where
Are the biggest lotteries in life to bare
Some whine and call this fate unfair
Forming a victim's face to wear
Yet choosing a positive attitude that cares
We can succeed where others do not dare.

An Aged Native Man

My mental conflict influenced my trekking off course.
Yet I felt a divine hand was at the source.
Went past red rock and mesas never seen.
Not recognizing landmarks for this human being.

A thin smoke line spiraled beyond the bend.
Contact, a message, surely a person did send.
Parked my ATV beside a skinny gray mule.
Saw an aged native man sitting calm and cool.

"Rest your knees my friend, warm yourself by the fire."
He sat cross-legged, peaceful pose, no urgent desire.
"I lost my way somehow, left my friends at the bar."
"Doesn't matter," he said, "wherever you go there you are."

"There's a secret to becoming ninety nine," he stated with verity.
"Just don't argue with people, gives me my longevity."

"I doubt that's the cause", I said with frowning curt brevity.
"You make a good point," he nodded with smiling clarity.

This white-haired guy had sure got me there.
I believe he had more life lessons to share.
I asked if he would tell me his wise living rules.
He agreed to relate his lifelong serenity tools.

With the suddenness of a broken shoelace he began,
"You will feel good completing a job with your own two hands.
One man's trash is another man's treasure.
Don't confuse truth with your lust for pleasure."

"Don't spend your life finding fault in others,
Righteousness lacks meaning unlike kindness toward brothers.
Without free will there's no accountability,
Any different belief permits every possibility."

"Do not complain about that which you permit.
Integrity is being okay with your life's conduct in print.
Your work will keep you alive from nine to five.
It's what you do after five that'll make you thrive."

"You don't always know who you know, knows.
The stranger is a friend you just don't yet know.
You don't know what you don't know, that's why you don't have.

It's our responsibility to create our own personal salve."

"It's better to say something than nothing at all.
Just accentuate the positive, avoid a verbal brawl.
Lovers and liars will gameplay in our head.
If we knew our future we wouldn't get out of bed."

"What doesn't get measured doesn't improve.
Abuse beats unused and time will then soothe.
A goal of any kind with no time deadline,
Is a fanciful wish with no risk on the line."

"With every choice we make we forfeit something.
We must embrace losing and endure the sting.
The most precarious of all is the marriage decision.
Blessed are those who keep focused and lack peripheral vision."

"Expecting fulfillment in relationships will fail,
You'll end up hurt, holding grievance, with your love life in jail.
Prioritize harmony, not being right, is life's craft,
Feels so good when your gut aches with a belly laugh."

"People are different, no one is ten out of ten.
Some like to explore while others stay close to the den.
Dusk swallows the day and dawn conquers the night.
So while we live, let us live, and live right."

Unhooked he didn't look as he taught his life's tale.

It was now up to me the course I'd set sail.
I tipped my hat to this stranger for telling me what he knows.
Convinced of dire consequences if I believe anything goes.

An Unknown Hormonal Urge

As I laid on my couch in a cozy repose
I recalled my youth on those Saturdays of old
It was that innocent time before puberty began
Where everywhere we went we ran and we ran

After morning chores we'd go knocking on doors
Asking neighbours for spare beer or pop bottles they'd stored
We'd take any apple baskets too we'd pleadfully dare
Pulling the red wagon full of our salvaged ware

Then off to the corner variety store and local farmer's market
Selling our cargo hoping for sixty cents as our target
Next we'd cash in and get eight packs of cards to split
The last twenty cents for an orange Crush and potato chips

Before Fleer, Upper Deck, and Donruss were alive
It was only Topps and O Pee Chee that made our heroes thrive

Impatiently eager we'd find some quiet outlet
Then carefully peel open each pack to see who'd we get

Football, hockey, and both baseball leagues.
Individual players, teams, all stars, checklists, and rookies
Sharing the chewing gum inside which came as a treat
Such shiny and colourful cards, they were just so neat

Looking for Mantle or Maris, any Yankee player was great
The 'Rocket', Hull, and Howe shooting as they skate
Faloney, McDougall, and Etcheverry were my favourite
No basketball, otherwise getting Cousy and West would be basic

Eventually got the whole set of the NHL six teams
The same for the CFL which was always my dream
The baseball set had just too many players and stars
Never did get them all before my interest turned to cars

So much fun too, at recess and before school
Trading with others, there was nothing more cool
"Got 'im, got 'im, got 'im, need 'im, got 'im, need 'im"
We all knew who had the rarest cards and we hung around him

Our passion was to complete the set and add to
our deck
We played to win, tucking away our best cards
we'd checked
Topsie's, flipsie's, knock downs, and closie's for sure
Looking for new lads we could play with and lure

Then one day after an unknown hormonal urge
I felt why Mature, Ladd and Granger always had
this urge
They'd fight and swashbuckle for Seymour and
Simmons
I felt I now understood why these legends kissed
women

One recess day those double dutchers I ne'er
noticed before
Held all my attention beyond collecting sport cards
galore
Hence with a shout to all I let the cards fly,
"It's a free for all..., SCRAMBLE," was my wave
goodbye.

Published in *Latchkey Lyricality,* Poetry by Members of The
Ontario Poetry Society, pg. 180-181, September 2016

A Warning Or An Invitation

Been awhile since I had
a girl interested in me.
No coquettish smile, no flirt
directed my way.
No anonymous note nor
clandestine Valentine card.
No unexpected conversation
unrelated to our work, from
a female colleague.
Not even a special twinkle or soft
hand on my shoulder,
from a skin revealing waitress
as she took my order.
Must be my age now, grey
hair, just doesn't cut it.
Maybe a facial wrinkle too, actually
maybe two or three, and a
more bull legged gait.
Sure, possibly wiser now,
but physically don't offer
that youthful spicy taste.
So it was I thought,
accepting that it is
what it is, until

that fortuitous night, an
unplanned rendezvous with
a gal I've day and night dreamed about,
to kiss.
It was a charitable event, a
truly good cause.
Perhaps the atmosphere made her
generous, desiring to give
and not take.
Whatever her motive,
her eyes gazed at mine,
held them and followed, there
was no mistake.

Five and a half feet tall,
thirty years younger than I,
with wavy brunette hair, and
an olive complexion that matched her
joyful jade eyed vision.
Elegant, sexy, confident, a
long thigh slit up her white gown,
next to nil bling, and a low
décolletage for a voyeur's caress.
I couldn't believe it.
An unexpected pleasure, yet
I was doubting, was
she really eyeing me?
What'd I have to lose?
I was so green at this
a 'no' from her wouldn't
make me blue.
I held her sight and then
desire dared me to smile,
subtle, yet clearly,

having faith too
in the verity of her blaze.
For certain, the corners of her
full rose lips upturned, they parted
and she returned a beam.
So mysterious, intoxicating,
a whispering call.
She vibrated magnetic allure.
I felt the titillating arousal of
piloerection.
Such a startling portent.
Was this a warning
or an invitation?
My hearts mind was afire.
She separated from her group,
and walked out alone onto
the terrace.
Before I had connected my
thoughts, my feet had shadowed
her and emboldened by passion,
I joined her at the balcony.
At once she turned toward me,
I swallowed.
Up close I recognized her now.
I'd seen her before, many times,
amongst the city of employees,
within our corporations' doors.
Over the past year, in
the hallways at work,
we'd nodded, smiled, exchanged
a friendly greeting, without
ever stopping to talk.
Didn't want to lurk or
be a jerk, feared more

she would reject my approach.
I lived a fantasy after each
serendipitous contact,
imagining being with her, hearing
her laugh softly and lightly,
brushing against my side and..., then
back to work.
It was a mental emotional,
virtual affair.
As though we both knew
we craved each
other, and each moment
of brief meeting, I sensed our
look lingered, our walk tarried,
expressing a surreal
intimacy wherein we moaned an
insatiable ardour for the other.
True, I thought, her age
compared to mine,
could be that of a daughter,
but rationalized that perhaps her
own attraction was maybe to a man
aged like a father.
I deleted these thoughts
replacing them with, "why not?"

Computed that she was
interested in me, at
least that was my
wanton fantasy.
I then repressed all
such thinking, for
it dulled my actions,
having learned that

analysis can lead to
paralysis, so no
thank you to that.
I longed for that which
I thought I could not have,
and now, she was here beside me,
moving nearer, a foot apart,
her hand resting just an inch
from mine on the railing,
her bosom rising and falling,
quicker, our combined concupiscence
fervently exposed.
I stood gripped in my view of her,
those full, red moist lips,
unblemished face, I
couldn't stir.
I felt awkwardly comfortable,
like a poem waiting to be rhymed.
Another step she took, and
then her fingers touched mine.
She called me by name,
in a clear melodic soprano voice.
Of course she knew me, and
I knew her, also by name
though I didn't speak it.
I just kept looking at her visage
and smelled her warm aromatic
breath, touching my face
I felt precariously on the
brink of an enchanted threshold.
Her hand reached out
and stroked my cheek,
and then, all reason
was gone.

Didn't matter now
who saw or who would talk.
We melted our lips
together.
Our tongues sought to entwine.
My arms wrapped around
her body,
squeezing her breasts to my chest,
she came even closer,
into me, all of her.
I could feel the mutual
rapture of our wanted embrace.
The invitation I took,
though still a warning may it be.
I hungered solely for her company.
Weeks and still months later,
we unabatingly meet,
so discreet.
Perhaps it is the stealth,
the naughty, that sustained the
kindling of our passions' palpating beat.
Amidst the stresses of life,
debt, deadlines, doldrums and drudgery,
we continue to covertly exchange
our cozy, tender, ardent, and
yes, prurient amused glances
of planned 'thee and me' encounters
to become one.
Shilly-shallying I unabatingly played,
as I privately remained unconvicted.
Perhaps I had ignored a warning,
only to be invited to a perilous
pleasure, toward my own
perdition.

Believe I'll Find

We all want someone to 'stand by me'
We all just want true love indeed
We all really want another's loyalty
We all want that honest friend we need.

I had helped them out so many times
Rescued them from mistakes and their social crimes
Sacrificed my own advance to achieve
This never seemed enough, no reprieve.

When I was down and out and in desperate need
Thought they'd be there with help as agreed
Their excuses for absence became my damnation
I now accepted this real expectation.

Their heart was good as was their intent
But their spirit was weak and selfishly bent
No truth to one good turn deserves another
That what goes around comes 'round to the other.

Forget this karma that bad deserves worse
Fact is, we just wanna witness this revengeful curse
Life's unfair to all so it's fair to all brothers
Gotta stop thumb sucking and pouting forever.

Thus I asked another to dance with me
I received a frown and she said laughingly
"No thank you", said she, "Not with you".
"Don't want to dance with someone like you".

I don't thrive on rejection, that's for sure
That line was only one opinion, now a blur
Their loss, not mine, I've made the attempt
Not gonna dwell on that rude comment.

Cause there's plenty of fish out there in the sea
And what's most important is my belief in me
So I'll continue to seek and believe I'll find
That partner who thinks with a likeminded mind.

Dancing to Victory

Do I matter to her at all?
Does she ever even think of me?
I really don't know what happened
Laugh'n and lov'n one minute
Then cry'n alone in the freez'n cold

Physical touch is my primary love language
Affirmations and deeds of service are her's
Never a 'no' to her reno requests
Easily applaud her talents unceasingly
Her beauty surpassed only by her generosity

However, I'm not the target of her kind donations
Not even on her radar to please
My heart saddens watching a woman's caress
Stroking her man's back standing together
A silver screen kiss has become my jealous bliss

Do this, don't do that,
I wasn't enough like…, whoever
Seemed everyone liked my jokes,
My silken wit, my sense of humour
She alone somberly tolerated my quips

You know how it goes
Rules without relationship
Cause rebellion
And so I try to stop catering
Discontinue my perceived sacrificial compromise

I accept she doesn't love me
I understand she doesn't dislike me
It's just the barren indifference
The apathy, the lack of expressed empathy
It's a killer on Valentine's Day

Okay, so now what?
Pout, have a pity party for Pete?
Change my scene, seek a new tasty green?
No thanks, my name's sake means rock
Thus I'll keep hope'n, trekk'n, and rock on

We don't verbally fight and rarely argue
I just go along, agree, hold her to no accountability
Mine is not to question why
Mine is but to do, then die
That is, do according to what I believe

No use asking others what they'd do
Get as many 'right' opinions as sand in the sea
Need to know my own priorities
Why I do what I do?
Being treated indifferently, is just my zoo

You see being loved, desired, and cared for
Comes second place to our children
Their health, security, dreams and desires
Outweigh my own self centered indulgent need

They're prioritized above my own narcissistic pleasure

So, I roll with the punches
Develop a rhinoceros hide
Grow duck feathered shoulders and back
Hone my comical communication, checking my pride
Then dancing to victory when she smiles at me

Everything Matters

Some say we're here for a good time not a long time
Some say life is short and we live on borrowed time
Some say we should do as we feel and live by our heart
Some say it's all over when death do us part.

So does it really matter what we say or do?
Does it really matter being Christian, Muslim or Jew?
Does it really matter if you work hard or not?
Does it really matter if you're humble or a snot?

We asked the children and here's what they say;
It matters that you brush your teeth and that you pray
It matters that you wear a smile and do your best
It matters that you run and play and sleep and rest.

It matters that you are sorry when you are wrong
It matters that you apologize when you've done wrong
It matters that you greet your neighbour and help them out

It matters that you're a good sport and don't whine or pout.

It matters that you hug and kiss each other goodnight
It matters that you make up before sleeping after a fight
It matters that you hold hands and serve one another
It matters that you forget the past and forgive your brother.

So when we look to the children and hear what they say
They've got it right and one day we'll pay
In the end there's a scoreboard laid out on a platter
Living bad or good counts, because everything matters.

False Evidence Appearing Real

Strange what we are afraid of
Yet we have all experienced fear
The dark, heights, crowds, even a family party
Can bring us to fright and tears

Coached to fret not and don't worry
For it only makes us more sick in the head
Our body too will ache and purge us
As we are gripped by this anxiety instead

Fear of failure often stops us
So we don't achieve our goals
Nor our desires and full potential
Beaten and crushed on life's shoals

We'd rather be inside the casket
Then publicly speak of the one interned
Palpitations, dyspnea, light headed and tremulous
We insulate ourselves watching our hopes burn

The secret is to feel that fear
But do the task anyway
We only get better by facing it
Only this keeps the monster at bay

Like the story of the village in the valley
Whose people feared that monster in the cave
No one ever dared near the mountain
All knew they'd be eaten then buried in a grave

Along one day came an adventurer
An upbeat, fit, and attractive lass
She couldn't believe these stories
Stunned by the villagers fear en masse

She turned on her phone's flashlight
saying, "I'll go and kill this beast"
She asked, "Who amongst you will come with me?"
No one moved to help her, standing alone was she

So she set out and found the cavern
Saw a shadow flash against a wall
She entered and looked about her
Then felt struck and began to fall

Now she wondered if she would be swallowed
Consumed by some unknown beastly thing
But heard voices and felt hands helping her
Saying, "Hey, welcome to our fun and partying"

They told her they had come here for years
Sharing ideas, yearning, and visions
Banished by the mayor of their village
'No dreamers allowed' was his scared decision

You see fear is a terrible prison
An acronym for false evidence appearing real
We must gather knowledge, courage, and wisdom
In so doing our true selves will we reveal

Fountain Of Youth

Woke up one day only to find
Had dropped some lift in his unfirm behind
His smiling wrinkles no longer looked neat
Have permanently now formed unsightly crow's feet.

Bent over just to pick something up
Had to rest his hand on his knee-"geez what's up"?
His forehead's grown larger and cranium more bare
His back, nose and ears found the missing hair.

Telling a story that they've already heard
Embarrassed - but not really, forgetting some words
Defending memories with, "Those were the days son"
No belief that the good old days are yet to come.

Critical of technology, no texting, no twitter
Unable to change an attitude of quitter
Forgot the ninth beatitude, complaining of aches
For blessed are the flexible as they'll bend, not break.

Ponce de Leon searched for the fountain of youth
It's not a cream, it's an attitude, that's the truth
Amazing we were all meant to work, love, and play
If you retire in one, you lose more than payday.

Try swimming or building, an adventure brave and bold
For it's when you stop playing that you really grow old
Avoid rockers, and lazy boys, those senior 'Geri-chairs'
Get excited by sights around you, not the vacant old stare.

Don't dwell on losses or mistakes you've made
Any deeper in that rut and you'd call it a grave
Defy GBS'S adage that youth's wasted on the young
Let history sing out the legacy you've won.

Glass House Living

I use cannabis weekly
and that's a certain fact.
But I've never shot up horse,
nor even snorted crack.

It's true I drink too much,
then sometimes say the wrong things.
But I've never been in jail,
nor had adulterous flings.

I'm thirty pounds overweight,
and I'm an absentee gym number.
But I walk my dog daily,
even in the cold days of December.

I'd never rip off a lemonade stand,
nor steal from any convenience store.
But no one declares all at customs,
and taking from large Corp's is my dutiful chore.

I'd never show too much cleavage,
nor squeeze into a skin-tight outfit.
But certain occasions warrant exposure,
and if I got it, I will flaunt it.

So we justify and rationalize, even a white lie,
as our negative judgments continue to grow.
We focus on the speck in another's eye,
ignoring the lumberyard in our own.

We need regular checkups from the neck up,
or forever prideful critic we'll remain.
For we judge and applaud our virtues,
by the vices from which we abstain.

GUTS

Don't we all just love adventure
and the thrill of that victory?
Yet we tend to only learn more
down on our knees while suffering.

Easy to be kind and giving
to our friend and good pal.
Try offering similar kindness
to our brothers broken in jail.

Cause it takes GUTS to take the high road
it takes GUTS to turn our cheek
it takes GUTS to forgive our neighbor
gotta Get Uncomfortable To Succeed.

Kinda nervous going to a funeral
and don't really know what to say.
It gives respect to those left living
we feel better at the end of day.

Want to lose weight and get leaner
means more protein and lower carbs.
Break and rip muscle in our workouts
will reward our self-esteem by far.

Become a Lawyer, a Doctor, an Actor
or a millionaire in business by thirty three.
You need to sacrifice, practice delayed gratification
takes strength of character in this microwave society.

So anything is possible if you believe it
and you can become the person you want to be.
Add zero doubt, elbow grease, and wise counsel,
plus a narrow snipers' focus, and true grit's certainty.

Healing Of Time

Going back to visit my folks
Home cooked meals, sharing old jokes
Hugs and kisses, gentle teases in kind
Warming the heart, comforting my mind.

But visiting the roots can be hard on some
Smells surface memories second to none
That loss, that fight, that pain returns
Paradise lost and relationships that burn.

Tragedies become lessened with the healing of time
Embarrassing moments forgotten with the healing of time
Failures and pain disappear with the healing of time
You can feel better with the healing of time.

No need to envy our happy friends
Celebrate their joy and learn from them
Don't criticize, complain or condemn the next guy
Seek to compliment, emulate, well at least try.

Develop a hide less sensitive to attack
So assaults and onslaughts roll over our ducks' back
Embrace the virtues of forgiveness to all
So tragedy plus time equals laughter for y'all.

Homo Sapien

Why you are
who you are
is key to examine.
Who you are
right now is
vital at present.
All this awareness
pales in comparison to
who you want to become.

You are not your history
nor are you shackled to your
character of the past.
You are not the beast
behaving by hormonal instinct.
You are not the
permanently spotted leopard.
Rather you are an
unknowing caterpillar now cocooned.

What stops your transformation?
It is not ignorance as you rationalize.
Laziness may contribute
but that's not all, that'd be a lie.

It is fear that imprisons your God given gift.
You forsake your growth for security.
Who you truly could be
remains buried.
You are more than you believe.

It's What We Finish

Anyone can start something
A diet
A workout routine
A marathon
A climb
A task
A book
A degree
A dissertation
A resolution
A commitment
A covenant
A marriage
And so on, and so forth
It's what we finish
That counts

Completing that what which we began
This is the muscle of character
The right stuff of heroes
The building blocks of self esteem
Bricks of perseverance,
Stamina, forbearance,
Longsuffering, hope,

Faith, forgiveness,
Passion, kindness
Responsibility, accountability
All built on a
Foundation of
Personal self-discipline
Held together by
The mortar of love
Towards mankind

Just Go The Right Way

Doughnuts or celery, it's your choice
Lie or speak truly, it's your voice
Watching shows of reality, night after night
Or live in the real world, and fight the good fight.

Avoiding the conflict because of the price
Run now for safety as it sure feels nice
Managed by fear depletes a man's soul
Courageous conversations are the only way to go.

You want their body so you'll say what you must
An Oscar performance to gain their trust
You remain involved, til you're satisfied
Justify your conscience that you've never lied.

Sex, power and money are icons of lust
We pursue them with passion until we go bust
Thirty years later we ask where we are
In nowhere land, eyes off the North Star.

So you just need to go the right way
That's it, just go the right way
If you don't that's not very clever
If you don't you'll be lost forever.

Life's Marathon Sprint

If you're on the wrong path, speeding up won't help
Making decisions at the peak of passion also won't help.
Having an atheist's creed in a foxhole, so too won't help.
In the end grabbing hold of your wallet, just won't help.

What to do when you haven't a clue?
"Regrets, I've had a few," just isn't true.
Chose that fork in the road, but whoever knew?
Wise counsel from one, beats listening to a loud crew.

Haste makes waste, but we worry to hurry
Must get it done quick, a mistaken flurry
We don't want to miss out, we're a harsh judge and jury
So the rose goes unsmelt, our priorities topsy-turvy.

Live For What You're Here For

Studied hard and became an engineer
Not for me but for my mother dear
Got married too, it just seemed right
It certainly pleased others, a welcomed delight

Got the suburban home, at preconstruction price
My spouse was happy it was so fine and nice
Yet restless I was, had no time to think
Started to calm my conflict with too much drink

Alfie wasn't the one to ask, he didn't know
Neither did the Jones' nor any average Joe
I just didn't want my last breath to be
I wish I'd been true to become my unique me

You've got to live for what you're here for
Live for what you're here for
You've got to live for what you're here for
Have courage to risk and free up thee

Quo Vadis? - a question to myself I rarely ask
Avoid this reflection with distractions and tasks
Yes I know the route to Bloor and Yonge
My GPS describes the way with her computer tongue

I tell Expedia where and when I want to go.
Even choose my comfort level and how fast or slow
Can plot the ten year strategic vision of our company
Choose the books I read and the associates I keep

Though once the long run is done, where have I gone?
Have I efficiently used my time or myself I've conned?
Amassed millions, wrote books, and awarded city gate keys
All matters not if my quest was other's to please

You've got to live for what you're here for
Live for what you're here for
You've got to live for what you're here for
Have courage to risk and free up thee

Live To Learn To Live

Learn as though you'll live forever
Live with passion and purposeful endeavor
Learn to avoid running with the herd
Learn to be known that your worth is your word.

Learn to enjoy the salty soft touch of an ocean swim
Live beyond moderation and fill your life's brim
Learn to overcome Auld Lang Syne's sorrow
Live as though there is no tomorrow.

Learn that faith in your love's quest will not perish
Live for her eyes that swallow and cherish
Learn that your life's conduct survives your death
Live for her look that still's your breath.

Learn to grow a hide that takes insults and laughs
Live to see her image painted on your aircraft
Learn to believe your heart 's wherever 's your address
Live to order another drink from that bar's beauty waitress.

Learn her name in her own language
Live neither like a 'veg' nor a savage
Learn what causes her to cry
Live to transfer your belief, certainly try.

Learn to hold no grudge nor any grievance
Live to smell her pheromone's erotic incense
Learn the secret that to live is to give
Live prepared to die in order to live.

Navigating The Ride

Be great to know then
what I know now.
Would have chosen the road
that showed me how.

With every choice I make
I forfeit something.
Want to minimize my loss
and maximize everything.

Always some butterflies
starting the race
Getting them in order
helps set my pace

Red, amber, green
and off I go
No impulse control.
This buck wants his doe.

Should have studied the trip
before launching ahead.
Courtship has gone.
Now, trial and error instead.

I navigating highways
of relationships and love.
Make dangerous decisions
when push comes to shove.

Was too young with Devon.
I made a lane change quick
Ignored signal turns,
Shannon didn't stick.

Failing to negotiate the curve,
Jamie fell away.
Now roundabouting with Riley,
I experience the sway.

Nascar, Indie, and Dakar
challenge the nerves
But mistakes with your partner
Cause your course to swerve.

Despite my best laid intent,
plans go awry.
I now drive life wisely
to avoid the big cry.

No More 'Yah But'

You have to quit smok'n
'Yah but' I really like tok'n
You have to lose weight
'Yah but' carbs taste great
You have to get exercising
'Yah but' I'd rather be carousing

You gotta flush that 'Yah But'
Just flush that 'Yah But'
Rotten in that rut of 'Yah But'
Just no more 'Yah But'

Gonna start right now
Resolve to eat less chow
Take care of my Mae Wests
Inhale only air that's best
Now Move and flex my core
So life's no longer a bore

You gotta flush that 'Yah But'
Just flush that 'Yah But'
Rotten in that rut of 'Yah But'
Just no more 'Yah But'

You could do this
But your 'Yah But' is your biz
You could do that
But 'Yah But' is your iconic hat
So opportunity gets stolen
Because it's your 'Yah But' you're hold'n

You gotta flush that 'Yah But'
Just flush that 'Yah But'
Rotten in that rut of 'Yah But'
Just no more 'Yah But'

Numero Uno

Survival of the fittest as Charles would say
The evolutionary path, crush any who pray
Lots of muscle, and lots of money
Influencing words to grab your honey.

Anyways we know that might is right
Even if your babe may feel fright
What can the next guy do for me?
That's the focus, that's our plea.

So war continues, here and there
Inequality, despite calls to play fair
We must get ahead, defeat our neighbour
Not realizing we're in self-destruct danger.

For need can be satisfied, greed cannot
If we don't give, our spirit will rot
Now why curse the darkness, light a candle instead
A candle loses nothing by lighting another candle head.

We must not criticize, condemn, or complain
Seek to compliment, build a positive brain
Read that forehead of that person so spent

It says for all - make me feel important.

For you know, the secret of living is giving
Not take, oppress, nor stealthy misgiving
This is how we become number one
Numero uno - that's how the race is run.

Passion Is A Permanent Partner Pact

Got a call from a gal
From a memory past
Just a friendly hello
Didn't think it would last

We met for coffee
Seemed innocent enough
Yet I kept it private
Rationalized as fluff

Then one thing soon
Led to another
We reminisced and laughed
Then touched hands together

Now it's sex with the ex
In stealth, under cover
A wild steamy ride
Makes for exciting lovers

I really did try to end contact
Even didn't show for our rendezvous
Yet we both boomeranged our liaison
Lust, not love driven, for the union of two

If you think an old flame is nothing
Think again before you act
Just play'n, laugh'n, and lov'n, but
Know that passion is a permanent partner pact

Recognitionem

"There's a handsome guy",
I heard sweetly from the side
I reflexly looked to her voice
To acknowledge her approved choice

Luckily checked my smile.
Pretending disinterest all the while
For she wasn't talking to me
But to a guy near some tree

I'm in an audience now listening to a speech
The speaker mentions special people he's honoured to meet
Now I imagine my name being preached
Hearing one's own name, there's nothing more sweet

Talking to others amongst a strange party crowd
I only knew one other who certainly knew me proud
Hoping he'd boast about my most recent victories
I craved the interest of the nearby beauties

Started as a kid playing out in the backyard
"Look at me mom", "watch me play lifeguard"

Now it matters most where I stand as a bard
Seems I haven't developed much since my grade schoolyard

Perhaps I'm alone in this quest to be seen
Taken too quickly from the breast, an inadvertent wean
Joined with my identity conflict that crystalized as a teen
Together fueled my ambition to forever be preened

Maybe my state is exaggerated yet it's still good to know
That our foreheads broadcast a message to show
'Make me feel important' we trumpet to each other
It commenced at first breath, our call to our mother

For to be desired, loved, and be recognized
Trumps self-preservation in life to be prized
Suicide proves that such amorous recognition is befit
As baby's cry and grown men and woman die for it

Remember The Time

Time flies by faster than you know
Like the speed of toilet paper coming off of it's roll
We remember happy times with others' spent
Yet can't forget other memories that we regret

Life's losses lead us to lessons learned
It's not when we're winning that our heart's get turned
It's on our knees suffering the laments of our acts
That's when life's wisdom makes it's impact

Remember the time we first tasted a peach
Or screamed in horror when Dad had a leech
Remember the time your fall skinned your knee
But Mom's love and band-aid healed you pain free

Remember the time you laughed til you cried
Or cried for real when you injured your pride
Remember the time you scored your first goal
Or prayed your bedtime prayers for your own soul

Remember your first goldfish or that first pet
Or catching that big fish so Dad used the net
Remember the time you stole that candy
Or the hurtful surprise when first stung by a bee

Remember the time you cheated on a test
Or then felt shame because they called you the best
Remember the last time you could truly be tickled
Or the last time your playful love to another did tickle

Remember the first time you saw turquoise water
Or making love to that person whose body was hotter
Remember that time of proposal, of "I do"
Or the first time you wanted to then say "adieu"

Remember holding that child and those innocent eyes
And realizing how love compounds and multiplies
Remember that time you won that award
Or being rejected by a friend who just got bored

Remember the time your child did graduate
Or how you mistreated that sad blind date
Remember meeting death at that loved one's funeral
And hence the moral changes you made to be kind and not cruel

So on we go and aged we all become
But personal growth is optional, chosen by some
For we don't stop playing when we get old
We get old when we stop playing, or so I'm told.

Small Talk

It's not a bad thing, actually important you know
To just start conversing with people you don't know
It's friendly to discuss weather, snow, rain, or sun
Introductions, schmoozing, while we work our day's run.

Try, "McIlroy is winning," "Have you checked out the zoo?"
Or, "Is it barbecue weekend?", "You look sharp in blue."
We all need to do it, to ease tension and stress
Silently crowded together only worsens our mess.

We need to improve ourselves, mix with the crowd
Be encouraging and cheerful, no need to be loud
Apply Mercer's principles and accentuate the positive
Latch onto the affirmative and eliminate the negative.

So, "Did you hear about Bo and Ray as well?"
Answer, "As long as it's complimentary, please do tell."
Swallow gossip now and it ends right here
Redirect the subject over your chips and beer.

Dreams start as an idea, then mold into an act
We need to communicate to feel true intimacy's pact
Yes silence is golden and still rivers run deep
But speak uplifting words, and you'll harvest smiles to reap.

Temperature Temperament

They say we're controlled by our DNA
That what's seen is because of our heritable genes, aye!?
Yet what moves us most and realigns our coast
Is the awesome weather which influences us most.

Waste not, want not, is what we're taught
Protect our ozone before we're all caught
Our footprint too must grow smaller you know
We're all in this together it's not just for show.

"Chilly out", "freezing", "cold as hell"
So we converse elevating new floors and tell
"Gorgeous and sunny", "Hope it stays that way",
That's our usual talk as we ascend our way.

Say anything we want on an elevator ride
The talks the same as it helps us slide
Money, sex, politics, and religion don't speak
But temperature affects everyone, the brave and the weak.

Whether sweltering, muggy, humid, or too hot
Or thunder and lightning and hail storms distraught
Eventually a soft breeze and sunlight does shine·
A covenant rainbow is a God send divine.

The Protagonist's Antagonist

His reflection was fearful,
but he was not,
not this time.
He knew his goal.
He wanted his prize.
Breaking bondage is good.
He had tried before,
many times.
Tasted the bitter sadness
of loss and defeat.
He knew now,
the obstacle creating his conflict,
was his own fear.
Such angst paves avoidant conduct
leading him to despair,
to stop short of commitment,
totally.
He was the antagonist
to his heroic self.
Letting go of an old, acceptable, yet
incompetent habit.
Scary.
The novel way felt awkward.
The behavior wasn't trained.

However, practiced,
such new action rewards a better,
experience.
Well worth comfort's sacrifice.
Perseverance pays.
He acknowledged no victory
without enduring the struggle.
The war continues daily,
sixteen centimeters between the ears.
Fuelled by a ventricular pump.
Different battlefields.
Different prices to be paid.
With unknown treasures to celebrate,
but only if the good guy
doesn't run, doesn't choose flight.
Instead, stands disciplined,
and fights,
to win
for Him.

True Romance

The wonder of romance
Is a distant memory
Being wanted, desired,
Craved, admired, pursued
Positively anticipating
Their reaching out to you
The other give's their all
Anytime, anything goes
For your pleasure and delight
Solely and totally

Sounds amazing
Almost unbelievable
Does it exist?
What does it cost?
What is its half-life?
And is this really romance?
Looks like a one way highway
All take and no give
Appears to be more like
Unilateral narcissistic gratification

Still I've tasted it several times
Indescribable, wonderful experience

Sometimes for a night only
Sometimes several weekends
Sometimes for months,
Even a year, maybe two
Then poofffff, it's gone
Evapourated
Maybe a slight cosmic trace left
Maybe

So now I work,
I provide
I parent
I compromise
I dream
I fantasize
Imagination defeats reality
This I know
So too, passion trumps reason
This I'm aware

However, I've grown
Thus I won't be tempted
I won't be trapped
I have re-prioritized
Crystallized my raison d'être
Forget whatever was
Or whatever may have been
I just need to do
What I don't want to do
To get what I want

When I was a child
I thought and behaved as a child
Every day, every morning,

I re-focus, I set my stage
Prepared to fight, to win
Courage is a perishable skill
So I must always be prepared
Romance is love shared between two
Neither a noun nor an adjective
It's a verb when it's true

You Can Do It

What to do?
I know right from wrong
Since I've been eight
I really do
I want to do what's right
Such a price though
Forfeiting physical pleasure
Life's so short
It's tough too
Financial expenses
Relationship challenges
Work
Surely a little indulgence
Is okay
There are worse things to do
To help you get through
A peccadillo or two
I mean…, come on
It's venial
Still, it is wrong
Amazing how easy it is
To alter our belief
To justify our behaviour
Yet how difficult it is

To change our behaviour
To align with our belief
Yet sudden acute illness
Can become our saving grace
We are now invulnerable
To temptation
We no longer will
Covetous thoughts
Nor lustful acts
Brought down on
Our knees
We may even humbly
Pray
So why not
Dig our well
Before we are thirsty
And acknowledge
Another
Above our self
You can do it

What If?

'What if'? trumpets the dreamer
For them life is an adventure
Limitless possibilities

Not so the worrier
For them 'What if'? cries
Apprehension and impending doom

Obsessing over past negatives
Reliving their embarrassment
Feeling the angst of some ridicule

Fretting over possible future failures
Living and suffering the terrible event
Though it's never happened

Dwelling, rethinking, and ruminating
Becoming mentally incontinent
Soiling their day

Rumination doesn't equate with reflection
Nor to contemplation nor thoughtful analysis
It does not prepare the mind

Neither is insight gained nor are lessons learned
Instead neurotransmitters are burned up
Necessary for our future mood stability

We must be unfaithful to rumination
Block it, snap it to stop
Distract oneself through immediate positive action

A mantra with 108 beads helps
'Om mani padme hum'
Happiness to all sentient beings

Or embrace Matts words
And do not worry about tomorrow
For tomorrow will worry about itself

You and I

A Not So Ugly Ducking

Her siblings saw her as
the black sheep of the family.
Yet she never gave up hope that
one day she'd be the dark horse.
Trying to assert her opinion in
this nest of vipers, she heard their
assertion about her, that a leopard cannot
change its spots, that she was
as mad as a march hare, and
they cautioned each other to not
get her roaring mad, or they would
be badgered to death as payback.
So smug they were with their judgement,
snug as a bug in a rug.
She was clearly the fly in their ointment.
A bee in their bonnet.
If they didn't attack her directly, she knew
her conduct was always the elephant in the room.
Any display of sympathy to her plight, they
expressed with crocodile tears.
Even her own mother in her spurious defense
was like a wolf in sheep's clothing.
Her father's statements of support were
weasel words.

Truly within her own family she felt
like a fish out of water.
She was as strange and rare
to them, as hen's teeth.
Eventually she stopped talking, couldn't
open up.
Wouldn't respond to chides of
"Has the cat got your tongue?", or
"I guess you can lead a horse to water,
but you can't make her drink,"
or, "Why don't you just get off
your high horse?"
She didn't need to be a fly on the wall
to know that curiosity killed the cat.
She was always their discussed topic.
Defenseless, a lame duck.
Like a lamb led to the slaughter.
She was tired of being in the dog house.
They wouldn't hear her reasoning, nor
her pleas to hold their horses.
Even if they did, it'd be a kangaroo court.
So she left.
Cold turkey.
She needed time to think, search,
plan.
She made a bee-line for the corner pub,
and ran straight as the crow flies
to the 'The Pig and Whistle'.
Drawn like a moth to a flame.
In the past she'd been quite the night owl,
drowning her sorrows in liquid courage,
accused of drinking like a fish.
Grinning like a Cheshire cat, the bartender
slithered over like a snake.

"I see the chicken has come home to roost",
he tempted.
Vulnerable, she was, yet she resisted.
She couldn't let her life go to the dogs.
She wouldn't let her past mistakes be
the albatross around her neck.
Now was the time to separate
the sheep from the goats.
So she left, again.
Determined that there were
halcyon days ahead for her,
refusing to allow her
family and their criticism, to be the
tail wagging the dog.
She reasoned as well though,
that she wasn't innocent.
She forgave herself and then, she
forgave her sisters, brothers, mother, and father.
She was determined.
She was focused upon making amends too.
Time to pony up.
Yes, she was committed to improve.
She would go the whole hog.
No more being scattered, nor running
around like a chicken with its head cut off.
She had a goal, a quest.
She would become as sly as a
fox, and wise as an owl.
She had mentally crystalized her life's swan song.
Now she would fuel her faith with action,
though recognizing that the best laid
schemes of mice and men
might go awry.
True she might find herself barking

up the wrong tree,
but if a dog she is to be,
then she embraced being a dog
who is a man's best friend.
This kindness and loyalty,
she now desired to live.
And with that decision,
she was happy as a clam at high tide.

A Slice Of Life

A welcoming sting accompanies the initial burning stab
Only a dull hurt experienced as the blade slices
Analgesically distracted by observing
The bright red blood ooze and stream out
A crimson viscous fluid
Syrupy, dripping and draining

It warmly paints and bathes my thigh
Replacing my intolerable pain of emptiness
With a pseudo-illusion that I am alive
Such ironic mental alchemy
Transient calmness and false peace
Carving its tattooed scar of self-loathing

Why this time?
Why now and not two days or weeks ago?
No idea
However, I know I am hurting
Because I do feel angry
I've learned that connection

I morph these feelings quickly
Being hypersensitive to experience rejection

Recognized consciously or not
Always my invisible fifty feet antenna are
On the lookout for any signal of abandonment,
Ridicule, put down, dismissal, or criticism

For where there is smoke
I will interpret a bonfire of unwantedness
Then in a micro second reflex
My poignant emotional pain transforms into rage
From the assault I've often wrongly perceived
Nevertheless I impulsively strike back

Not always with a cut to my skin
Burning works too
Or head banging the closest wall
Perhaps punching my face
Or clawing my skin
Even plucking out my eyebrows and eyelashes

The destructive options are endless
Smashing plates, slamming a door, trashing the computer
Another personal signature hole in the dry wall
Or an irresistible urge to get inked or maybe pierced again
I can choose intoxication with alcohol or escape with cocaine
Regretfully spew serrated vitriol at my partner's heart

Possibly clean out the fridge with my binge
Then damage my enamel with a purge
Withdraw, hide in bed with extra pharma sedation

My fatigue and headache intensify
Whatever defensive offense I choose
Engagement of the dirty deed trumps all censors

Then, my guilt convicts me
Alone with my damning compunction
Pondering why do I even live
Yet, I hear a faint whisper of hope
I can learn to improve, truly get better
Forgive myself and defeat this biological
dysregulated disorder

It's not necessary to bask in resentment
Towards others nor to my own personal affliction
I will become responsible for my choice of reaction
Accept and commit to mindfully implement
Healthier self-soothing strategies
And never, ever, give up

Gregg

He was named Gregg - with three g's
A smiling friendly guy who liked to please
Strikingly handsome, desirous to most women
He couldn't say "no", creating his own prison

Yet it wasn't sex that turned him on
Being craved was his real love song
Physical contact he neither needed nor sought
Pursuit of others approval was his lot

He did favours for all around
For friends and strangers he generously gave abound
Bolstering his fragile self-esteem, countering self-doubt
From accolades of recognition as he awaited their shout

Detested confrontation, avoided any waves
Didn't like tension, only cowardly opinions he braved
Nurturingly conditioned from an emotionally upheaved upbringing
He was the glue, the family's ambassador of peace keeping

Thus he lived, precariously balanced on the fence
Until having children he realized his offense
He disagreed with many tolerated views
Decided to change, paid enough of 'should' dues

Now parenthood required love, sacrifice, and learning
A popular vocation professionally practised by a select yearning
Knowing that example is a good teacher for our progeny
They will do half of what we do right but all we wrongly do certainly

So he sought counsel, therapy for his dismay
Understanding his character more and improving to this day
Set boundaries to live and love but protecting his self
No longer felt bored or lost, erased his obsequious self

Fibro

Was punctual and always stayed late
and was the first to arrive too.
Held higher standards than the rest
and perfection was her temperamental aim.
Rigid opinions on the "How"
and barely tolerated another's view.
Knew she was more right than her peers
so alone she performed, without company.
Such accomplished workload did cost her,
adding two stones in adipose she bore.
Then came a merger, really a takeover,
and thus overtaken was she.
New authority didn't tremble nor fear her
nor adhere to her spoken word or advice.
She had been too strong for too long.
Now discarded like a cigarette butt.
No more brow control over colleagues.
Perceived unjust treatment from above.
Resented this undeserved brush off.
Never learned to let it go.
Insomnia, aches and tenderness
in more than eighteen body places at least.
Depression became her mood state
as no more recognition nor reward did come.

Anger built an internal hailstorm,
and the myalgia intensified still.
So the holes of Swiss cheese lined up.
Just took one more reprimand to collapse.
She could not take another onslaught towards her,
and so immobilized and disabled she did lapse.
Tried to return to the front lines,
but she was disabled, her pain would not allow.
Now only misery and agony are her workmates.
Trapped by silent bitterness as
her sole companion as well.
No one understands, no one believes.
If one cannot live with oneself,
one certainly cannot live with one's neighbour.

Insomnia

Why can't I sleep?
Every evening I have only one
glass of the fruit of the vine.
Regular morning exercise and
I'm only four kilograms over weight.
I'm not recreating with any
street drugs, nor am I
napping during the day time.
All caffeine is consumed before noon,
neither snacks nor fluids
two hours before retiring.
My thyroid 's okay.
No sleep apnea.
Even got a new
posturpedic and flip it
every three months, plus
heavy bedroom drapes keeping
the darkness in and noise out.
Wear loose fitting PJ's
or my birthday suit only.
Yet still I frequently awaken
during the early morning hours,
resting ever so lightly, though
only minutes after becoming supine

I'm out.
No trouble shutting the mind
down.
Not anxious, nor fretting.
Apprehensive about nothing, so
sleep is easily induced, however,
lasting for only an hour at most.
Then starts the tossing
and turning, the watching the
clock, accompanied by a loud inaudible
'tick-tock'.
Why?
Why can't I get eight hours of restful
undisturbed sleep?
Been feeling a little
more irritable lately too,
and my appetite and motivation are
down.
Even my libido is
off, and getting emotional
watching television commercials.
What's that all about?
I haven't even played hockey
for the past two weeks.
What's keeping me
up at night?
I knew though, I
really knew.
I didn't want to admit it.
I'd rather not be conscious
of the reason, but
the rapid eye movement nightmares,
their unconscious content had
exposed my soul.

My integrity I had
compromised.
My values I had
contradicted.
I couldn't get away
with it.
No one knew,
no one, except me.
I knew what I had done.
The pain I had
caused, the selfish
gain I had bought.
This shame and
guilt were my
insomnia's origin.
No longer could I
sleep on the sweet pillow
of a clear conscious.
Being down was keeping me
up.

Mirror Mirror On The Wall

Ordered by the court to get some help
Pled guilty to the crime but silently yelped
Really didn't believe he was at fault
Believed the justice system wasn't worth their salt.

Explained to his "shrink" the way he saw it
Had a right to those expenses, seemed only fair to profit
Not for others of course as that'd be wrong
He continued to indulge his entitlement song.

His captivated wife felt like his deserved utility
A chattel, an accessory, to boast his virility
He owned more skin products then her as well
His well-coiffed mane was better groomed than his belle.

He'd achieved economically, though his birthright did assist
Claimed too an expertise in music he did insist
And proficient in squash and handball he did tell
His spoken deeds of prowess could not be quelled.

Even stated a milestone of walking at age eight months
Placed in gifted classes he said, not with the regular runts
Unbeknownst to him, his rant had an irritating effect
His therapist suffered with formication, neck hair erect.

Was clear he required excessive admiration
Any reality feedback was perceived as a damnation
Known for his grandiose self-importance and arrogant citations
Viewed being drawn accountable as others envious castration.

Hearing the victim impact stories of his acts
Felt deflated and misunderstood by these quacks
He defended his talents as unique and superior
Unwilling, at least unable, to listen with an empathic ear.

His history did reveal a critical rejecting father
Who also was often absent or didn't care to bother
So too an emotionally abused mother by his dad
Yet she perpetually praised him as a very special lad.

So as the young boy grew, excuses were made
"It wasn't his fault, he didn't lie, he was swayed."
Mom bent the rules for him which he came to accept
And dad wasn't there, or viewed him with contempt.

He was brighter than the average bear for sure
Handsome and street smart, definitely not a boor
Thus doors opened for him and society promoted his climb
He expected such recognition, a legend in his own mind.

Often wrong though never doubting, very self-assured
Would occasionally feel uneasy, his unconscious being lured
Briefly thinking sadly of his family, his past
Then reflexively pursued more financial gain, his thoughts recast.

Incredulous for him that he be brought to such an account
Couldn't believe he was wrongly caught, demanding a recount
Angry at the media's word that he was a slime
They were all just mediocre, not like him, so prime.

The sessions continued, but difficult to reach the core
Attempts at intimacy, trust, self-esteem conflicts were explored
Though he never did own true personal responsibility
Feeling forced to attend, he maintained his character disability.

For he had paper thin loyalty even to his "friends"
Was indifferent to both injustice and its victims
He saw himself as a comic book superhero

Whose identity he'd never hide, that'd be 'sicko'.

He didn't really love himself, didn't seem to care
He loved the adulation and praise of those faked by his flare
Calculating and crafty, he secured power for continued praise
Defied authority through subtle disobedient manipulative plays.

His depravity was finely disguised as a paragon of virtue
Took advantage of people in need, showed false favour, so untrue
A few saw beyond his charade, his underhanded schemes
Knew his real vindictive nature, his plot to make them scream.

When he'd served his time and therapy was no longer mandated
He terminated such treatment with an expectation to be reinstated
He had enough funds, and duplicit favours he'd collected
Got himself a new wife, private clubs, hence was re-elected.

Though attired loud and proud in his suit outside
He carried a fragile self, quite a vulnerable pride
Disabled to reflect on life's lessons, unable to be taught
Conflicted by rejection and specialness, nurturingly bought.

Painfully True

She was having some severe headaches
much different than before.
Not in the temples, but her upper neck and scalp,
'Could this be something more?'

It'd been a year since she had
a complete physical and CT.
An MRI would've been better
Surely then the doctors would see.

The neurologist seemed dismissive,
he didn't understand, just didn't get her.
What if it was a tumor or an aneurysm?
She was confident that he wasn't sure.

Others had died either with their symptoms
overlooked
or simply not taken seriously.
Just a week ago in fact her
cousins' friends' neighbor had passed mysteriously.

She knew something was wrong.
Already she had two other specialists booked.
She was tired of living with this pain,
though more annoyed by others rolling eyes looks.

"You're really a worry wart,
you know it's all in your head".
"You just need to cowgirl up,
quit complaining, get yourself out of bed".

Easy to say, they didn't comprehend.
They criticized, they didn't know.
They weren't words of a friend.
They were condemnations of a foe.

But what if?
What if they're wrong?
She knew that they were.
Her energy was ebbing, she was no longer strong.

Now she can't really cycle,
neither run nor swim.
She can't intensely work out,
gave her membership up at the gym.

What if she has a spell,
lost consciousness and fell?
She could suffer even further calamity
her confidence thinned to a shell.

For she could fracture a hip,
a mandible or her wrist.
It could happen easily,
She couldn't take that risk.

What if it occurred when she drives?
An accident pray God forbid.
Not only herself, but others could be hurt,
even die, so no driving she did.

Even shopping for groceries, or
going to church, a party, or out for dinner.
You name it, she couldn't do anything.
She'd become a loser, not a winner.

She'd be so humiliated, so embarrassed,
to have such an episode witnessed.
She really must stay indoors,
isolating herself was for the best.

She'd developed that one eyed
expression of defeat- "I can't".
Yet this pain and dizziness was so severe that
it was exhausting to move, her breath was a pant.

She'd worked hard all her life.
She didn't ask for this state.
She wanted to get better
be a contributor and create.

After so many M.D.'s that she'd seen, and
being prodded, probed, needle pricked and
scanned,
they concluded with finding only a minor
abnormality,
saying further investigation was unnecessary, was
banned.

Now she's sent to a 'shrink', to check this out.
Who wouldn't be depressed as she could do
nothing anymore.
Her family and friends have left her by now,
having their last laugh behind closed doors.

Suffered a blood clot in the calf of her leg,
and a two month infection after her fourth
spinal tap.
She'd only taken the narcotics as prescribed by
doctors,
and only used benzo's if she anxiously felt trapped.

The Psychiatrist said "yes" and "no" that it was all in
her head.
"No", if it meant that she was faking or making
it up.
"Yes", that it meant chemically produced pain,
when stress had overfilled her mind's coping cup.

The dizziness too he said
got processed the same way.
He assured her that she wasn't malingering
nor that she wanted this sickness to stay.

He told her the pain and dizziness were real
as real as the black chair they both could see.
However, the minimal abnormal findings to date,
couldn't explain her symptom frequency and
intensity.

He said that psychological factors were causing
her malaise.
He stated that she consciously didn't cause nor
want this illness.
However, he said the unconscious mind did control
this sustained ongoing pain, syncope and dizziness.

Then he said that if she didn't believe in this concept,
that her dulled mobility would cause her further distress,
and that she'd become addicted to pain and anxiety meds,
and that she'd potentially be injured from more medical tests.

Defensively she stated that she only did what the doctors ordered.
She didn't like taking meds nor being unable to function.
She didn't use street drugs nor drink alcohol either.
Asserted she wanted to get better, not undergo extreme unction.

Patiently he repeated that he believed her words true.
He explained neurotransmission, underlining unconscious power.
Said that what he was about to tell her would be difficult to hear.
His prescription caused conscious disbelief, a reflex to cower.

Pressing on he affirmed that her symptoms did remain,
by unconscious desire for affection, attention, being looked after,
from people around her that wouldn't otherwise be forthcoming,
and her symptoms falsely promised this faster and longer.

Yet suffering this disability also allowed
a socially sanctioned inability to work,
plus avoiding certain life personal responsibilities.
He emphasized the etiology being where the
unconscious lurks.

She couldn't believe this.
His words angered her so.
It still sounded like her fault.
He said "no", "for some that's just how it goes".

Now her task was to come off this analgesic patch.
No more codeine products, no relatives of 'pam'.
He asserted too, that she held anger inside, and
noted her dependent character, making her feel
slammed.

Now all else had failed.
She had nothing to loose.
His opinion was confident.
She did trust him, though her ego was bruised.

A program of physio to strengthen her balance
and gait.
Prescribing mindfulness therapy, and pain distress
strategies.
Arranging community nursing support, all
caregiver's looped in.
Adherence was paramount for her symptoms to
cease.

It wasn't a linear improvement,
and felt like 'snakes and ladders' she'd played.
She persevered with his kind competence,

experiencing increased comfort, while she also prayed.

Her memory returned, her focus, and her concentration and decision making too.
She wasn't out of the woods yet, but with daily training,
She could become well, this she knew.

Winner of 'Judge's Choice Award' in *Epic Proportions Contest Anthology - 2016*, The Ontario Poetry Society, Contest Judge - Bernice Lever

Purgatory Performance

It sounded good
She said she hoped to get better
She said maybe she could get well
She wanted to improve, no longer be depressed
She was going to try her best
You have to give her accolades
Her attitude was positive
She gave an affirmation of determined effort
Too bad though, it isn't enough
Hope, want, and try don't cut it
It's half hearted
Like walking into a lake on tip toes to mid thighs
It's easy to turn back when there's no genital dip
Like the Kamikazee pilot who flew twenty missions
He was involved, just not committed
Like a 'B' grade on an exam
It's not bad, it's just really not that good either
A purgatory performance
Not the mentality of any Olympian
"Maybe I'll medal", "Great to just qualify"
On the contrary, "I will win gold"
"I will set a new record"
"I don't know who will be second, but I'll be first"
"Bring it on, I will defeat everyone"

No limbo land thinking there
A mentality miles apart from 'try' or 'maybe'
A commitment of belief and will, trumps all
Unstoppable when backed with action
As faith without works is dead

Rise Up and Apologize

Time to say I'm sorry
Rise up and apologize
Don't wait, don't tarry
No 'if's', don't rationalize

Seems I'm one to never say I'm, sorry
Never admit that I'm wrong
Won't apologize for that hurtful comment
Believes it weakens and makes me less strong

Then I react, by stop talking to you
Cut you off with my silent angry sword
That was wrong of me to respond so
It's not the way of my Lord

Time to say I'm sorry
Rise up and apologize
Don't wait, don't tarry
No 'if's', don't rationalize

You see it's better to be hurt than to hurt you
Better to be lied to than to lie
Better to be deceived than deceive
Better to be denied then deny

It's better to be betrayed than betray you
Better to be assaulted than assault
Better to be cheated than to cheat you
Best to apologize for my own fault

Time to say I'm sorry
Rise up and apologise
Don't wait, don't tarry
No 'if's', don't rationalize

Serendipitous Salvation

I toiled with my thoughts
again thinking about myself,
what else of course but my favourite subject.
Fretting about bills to pay,
car windows aren't operating,
the fridge is croaking,
disgruntled about going into my job
which is boring at best,
sprained my ankle too so tennis is out this week,
feeling not loved enough, not needed enough
by my spouse and family,
and social obligations to attend a party and a wedding
making demands on me for my precious time.

Suddenly my ruminative sight becomes distracted
by seeing the scampering of a squirrel nearby.
Intimately I experienced an intuition, a hunch,
perhaps it was a vision,
certainly more than a portent or premonition
as all of these words conveyed too neutral or
too negative a description of this
positively glorious corporal tingling.
Well if Walpole could coin a word

for "fortunate happenstance" in 1754
then I could define my own neologism.
A divine nomenclature for such
a beautiful, supernatural, and personal
vibration of a wondrous pre-cognitive
event about to engulf me.

'Posipremonity' is the term,
a most positive premonition to be had,
indeed.

As my mood pinked
and a reflexive smile adorned my visage
a woman ambulated towards my bench.
She was slightly ataxic with a hesitant stumble
medium height and build, caucasian
early thirties with a pleasant face
amidst a nostril, eyebrow, and ear lobe piercings.
She sat beside me and congratulated
the sunny day and turquoise sky that
we were celebrating this day.
I agreed whole heartedly
as truly I had only then just noticed
the heavenly beauty that
had been showering upon me all this time.
I commented on her gait
inquiring if she were in pain.
She affirmed her discomfort
and proceeded to tell me her tale.

A cheerleader in high school and
at the top of her class academically,
she awoke one morning with marked malaise
very unlike her energetic self.

She missed three days of school and
then she turned as yellow as a lemon.
Aggressive hepatitis was the physician's diagnosis,
whose contact and cause
remains still a mystery.
It malignantly progressed
resulting in her necessitating
a liver transplant ten days later.
Medications, hospital bed,
weakness, and anorexia followed,
only for her body to reject the new organ and
additionally she developed B-cell lymphoma,
hence a second liver transplant.
Heavy steroids for three years
with resultant avascular necrosis led to
replacement of both her hips
and now her right shoulder is next.
Continued immunological treatment
with her orthopedic surgeon on speed dial.

Thus, "I walk kind of funny", she grinned.
"Even worse after a tonic and gin", she laughed.
"However, you would never know and
I'm danc'n because anything goes", she merrily
concluded.
Then she asked, "How about you,
how are you doing?"
Embarrassed about my earlier petty pensiveness,
yet realizing how I was so fortunate
I said, "I am doing very well".
"I am blessed and even more so now
to have met you".
"Your shared life is my serendipitous salvation".

Soft Place To Fall

The grey goose diluted
as the ice cubes melted, and
now it lacked it's tasty punch.
Just like my speech,
as the crowd went mild.
It's the corruption of the best
that becomes the worst.
Corruptio optimi pessima.

She was so genuine in a world
of fake smiles and white lies.
So soft, smooth and soothing,
lubricating my life's rocky road.
I had tried to curb my urge,
but was held hostage to my heat, and hers.
One loving heart sets another
on fire.

Her gentle smile, unsolicited touches,
her warm lingering kiss,
were sweeter than the comb's syrup.
Her love was honey for this bear.
There was a fork in the road,
a moment for me to decide.

She liked me, and had approached and
sought me.
She truly wanted my company.

I could be me with her.
Expose my fantasies, wishes
dreams and silly ideas.
No fear of ridicule, in fact,
even encouraged to speak,
about myself.
Likewise be vulnerable, and sad.
Yes, even cry over my painful losses.

I was older by two decades I guessed.
Could have been a colleagues daughter,
yet she really seemed to want me.
This beautiful woman desired me.
I'd been married now, twenty-five years and
running for office that was all but mine.
My children had launched, and were on their way
My wife's career too, had enjoyed independent
success.

My wife, my wife, what can I say?
Perpetually critical of my habits,
though not my work nor the income I made.
Irritated by my tapp'n fingers, rubbing my feet,
whistling not allowed, and denigrated my
attire too.
Besides repulsive comments and demands for my
change,
she treated her misophonia by abstinence from my
range.

Chided me for getting older, even the way I breathed.

Then came Judith, non-stop affirming me.
Actually laughing at my jokes, and conversing harmoniously.
Thus my rationalization began.
Over the hill is better than under it.
You don't stop playing when you get older,
you get older when you stop playing.
So I stepped beyond the precipice,
risking the abyss for these moments of bliss.

Such ecstasy, so wonderful, our stealth time of embrace.
Then months later while away on business
down on all fours behind closed doors, or so I thought,
my life got snap'd.
The pictures were released on every tube.
Surface scenes that would never be forgot.
I was done that was certain, position, family, and repute.
Crazy though, it didn't matter as long as Judith stayed afloat.

It doesn't matter that I grew the economy, passed bills
for senior benefits, education, and raised minimum wage.
It doesn't matter that I was in a loveless marriage,
working hard all my life, though my personal passion was caged.
My deceit to my wife, my affair of my heart,

lost people's belief in my morality and tore the party apart.
Like tennis I was defeated by a performance of love.
However, Judith was my soft place to fall, I didn't need a shove.

That Call In The Night

By this age there is not much I'm afraid of

There is nothing so blinding as fear anyways
Apprehension just handcuffs us from performance
Unnecessary hesitation and caution
Our idea, dream, goal, now escapes fruition
All around us becomes boundaryless, blurred
Out of our depth and deep in a fog
Yet experience, time, even a modicum of gained wisdom
These life gifts lyse our anxiety
I'm no longer afraid of that which I don't understand

Fearless, such a beautiful state of mind and body

The big 'C' can get any of us
So can an MI a CVA or an MVA
I'm not so myopic that I can't see this reality
Yet, peace, real contentment removes their growl
As well that roar of uncontrolled compulsive behaviour
Driving me toward secret unhealthy conduct, has ceased

Melted away into a shallow puddle
Like a snowball on a summers day
May I now walk the earth full of heaven's wonder
Become a water walker

But really I've fooled myself, I'm enacting the ostrich delusion

The truth is, there is something that frightens me
The mere shivering thought paralyzes me, sidelining my play
Without asking it waves a tsunami of horror terrorizing my core
An intolerable image that pummels a somasthetic torture
The hollow emptiness, the agonizing longevity of loneliness
The relentless pain, knifing, and then crushing my heart
Spiraling my spirit down like an auger into a living hell
It could arrive as a knock or without wire
Forever forbidding a restful sleep ever again
To have to receive, that call in the night
Numquam mihi Deus meus sepelire

Love

Edified

I didn't care what they said
I knew how I felt
More so I knew what I believed
In my youth
I'd been naughty, not nice
Thus never was I alone
Just loneliness was my price
Still, such suffering
Served my edification
I learned that
It's death that gives
Meaning to life
For if we live forever
Nothing would be accomplished
As we are already
Great procrastinators
Ignorance, laziness and fear
Immobilizing us
Holding us back
However make no mistake
Fear is the dark king
Imprisoning our dreams
And so I wandered
Under my delusion of adequacy

Often with feral butterflies
Beating my daily breath
With intercostal pain
I had tried to influence
The stiff necked people
And learned that to argue
With others stubborn stupidity
Will surely bring about their win
For they have so much more
Experience at that level
So be it
Anyways it's better to err
By excessive mercy
Than by excess of severity
It is the unnoticed
Acts of kindness
That justifies life
So I make my mind
Into a fortress
Where no thoughts
Will enter unless
I allow it
Now I remember to
Resume my life's purpose
An adventure to chase
And someone to love
Then to live to spend
Another day with that
Someone I love
And each day loving
Her more
Than the day before
Truly all is ephemeral
Except love

Give Thanks

It's okay if it ends now.
Quite fine if it stops here.
Never expected the joys I've had.
Children. Amazing. The best.
Their innocence, their laughter, their passion to breathe.

I have loved too.
Loved my children, and my mother.
They too have loved me in return.
Actually, perhaps first, they taught me.
I have loved a woman as well.
I think briefly she loved me.
Then unrequited was my love forever.

Still to tingle, obsess, crave our rendezvous.
Imagine her smile, natural, unforced, her gentle face,
her beckoning eyes, her rose moist lips to kiss.
She was beautifully formed and lovely to behold.
My pulse perpetually pounded in her presence.
So special she was.
So special she made me feel.
Once.

Only in love does participation surpass anticipation.
I've experienced this gift, this grace.
Many do not.

There is still love in me.
A gratitude of love.
Compelled to give thanks.
How?
Discover through sacrifice, self-discipline, and longsuffering,
by faith.
Who?
Totus tuus

I Just Love Her With All My Heart

I scanned the crowd and saw her there
Framed amidst her wavy black hair
Her light brown skin on shoulders bare
My gaze now fixed into a stare.

She turned toward the campfire light
A green eyed beauty dressed just right
Her eyes met mine and held them tight
Love really can strike you at first sight.

Then she smiled at me
Made me so very happy
I felt so 'fan-tast-ique'
Surely this is how heaven must be.

We left our own to join each other
No one could part our union asunder
More than the closeness of sister and brother
Our smiles and eyes caressing each other.

All others around now faded away
Heart pounding, lightheaded, starting to sway
Our lips came nearer, warm breath did say
We lovingly kissed and still do to this day.

I just love her with all my heart
No worldly force could pull me apart
A romantic attraction right from the start
I just love her with all my heart.

I'm "Lucky Joe"

She is great at her job and she knows it
Makes more than me but doesn't flaunt it
Turns guys' heads as she walks down the street
Full of confidence as she turns up the heat.

She's invited to the best of soirées
Soft smooth skin her age does betray
Enough cleavage to distract a focused talk
Men and women fix stares at her walk.

More than her curves she is loyal to me
Understands my needs, a consoler to me
Could have any guy who does better than me
Her devoted passion she focuses on me.

So I am Mr. Fortunate this I know
Count my blessings, I am "Lucky Joe"
I fuel her love languages to avoid hearing "no"
Doing my best to reap what I sow.

Not A Lonely Tale

It's humiliating to confess
but I have to, I must.
Actually only by enacting the compulsion
may I possibly be relieved.
So here it is, I'll say it
"I'm lonely".
It's true, I do feel more relieved
now that I've said it.
Just sharing this state of cerebro-cardiac being,
perhaps as well of my soul,
really does lessen my loneliness.
It's out there now,
I belong to the others who
also are embarrassed by
this admission of their life.
However, am I still lonely?
Really, it seems by this compelling confession,
especially to another,
I'm not feeling existentially alone anymore.
Now what?
Decisions.
Forks in the road.
Then like a fish, lured by the wobbler,
my eyes unconsciously turn to see

the wiggle.
Amazing.
Right leg forward, the ipsilateral hip dips
while the opposite buttock lifts.
One two, one two, right left, right left
Back and forth, back and forth.
My nystagmus of excitement
building like a tennis game of love.
Not even aware of my gluteal stare.
Next I'm laughing at myself.
From loneliness to love, or lust,
in a microsecond of time.
An instinctual reflex.
Is this testosterone's testimony?
My thoughts continue to drift and wander.
Freely associating in the realm of
heterosexual hypothesizing.
Women need to just be.
Men must do.
I'd be court marshalled by the
feminist squad for that ideation.
Yet, the evidence shows
that women outperform men,
if not at least equal them,
in just about everything.
The Natural Superiority
of Women says Montagu.
Women don't have to do anything
to be desired, craved, or
pursued by men.
Just be, with all their femininity.
Men can't just exist to be
desired, craved, or pursued
by women.

We need to produce,
at least provide some
reliability, perhaps a modicum of
consistent security.
Even to preserve the species, or have sex,
women need to just be,
men must get erect.
I'm not complaining.
That's a-ok for me.
Can't even imagine taking on
the trials and tribulations that
go along with the living
delights of being a woman.
They do more piercing than guys, but are
catching up to us in inking as well.
Not my taste.
Unblemished skin is best for me
except for scars which are
just tattoos with better stories.
They become pregnant too and
give birth to life.
Awesome.
They know how to let love in
and give love out.
So, again I ask, am I lonely now?
No.
Five senses to input information,
and still significant non-utilized gyri
to process the data.
An infinity of possibilities, therefore
I'm essentially never bored.
I am crying now.
Blissful tears.
No lakes of loneliness.

Alive.
Emotionally catharsed
I feel something special.
Did this exposure of my spirit
deliver me love?
I don't know.
I know I loved my mother, and
the simple truth is that
Moms are more important
than Dad's.
I know I love my wife.
Then my first child, I
experienced love multiplied.
With every child this intimate involvement with love
demonstrates its beautiful power of
compounding exponentially.
It's the greatest gift of life.
Learning love.

The Dinner Bell of Love

It's her smile that she cared
that was honey for this bear.
Still, if I were to embrace
her unfathomable pulchritude
I had to get out
of the shallow end.
For a wish changes nothing
yet a decision changes everything.
I only hoped
that she'd make for me
that special recipe.

I learned that
life is not all beer and skittles,
and finding that one,
so there would never be another,
may sound like pie in the sky.
However I had faith
that I'd find
that dish for the gods.
Thus cool as a cucumber
I walked into
the Amber Nectar pub.
A veritable feeding frenzy

it was, and I
was a 'yummy-man'.
My ears turned to
the lady in red
who winked and chimed
'eat, drink and be merry'.
I wanted dearly to
curry favour with
this vivacious vixen
knowing I must
chew the fat first
and simultaneously avoid
drinking like a fish.
Only then could I
chow down on
her mouth watering tasty-treats.
Yet though I felt
dramatically egged on
by this piping hot number
I knew she was not
my cup of tea
as she'd already lost the plot.
I figured the juice
wasn't worth the squeeze.
Furthermore, having assessed
that she was out to lunch
I knew I had to
make tracks quickly
or I'd lose
my own noodle
in the process.
Bummer, I really wanted to
curse, but cried
'cheese-whiz' instead.

Amongst the bakers dozen
of les jeunes filles
I was drawn to a new peach.
Her movements, her grace,
I was just confident
we were like
two peas in a pod.
I engaged her in conversation
however my nerves produced
a word salad forcing
me to eat humble pie.
Fortunately she welcomed
my awkward approach
and displayed a rare
milk of human kindness.
Although I thought
this green eyed gem
took the cake,
I discovered she had
a bun in the oven.
I exclaimed
'suffering succotash' and then
gently exited as
a gentlemen does,
as I wanted to
save my bacon and
not get myself into a pickle.

Taking leave, I was suddenly
tugged away by
Ms. Piss and Vinegar
who grabbed my arm
launching me onto the dance floor.
Her gyrations certainly

whet my appetite
and as she made eye contact
while eating a banana
she induced in me
salivating dreams
of a cream pie.
I justified that
I had heard it said,
that you are
what you eat.
So for example,
if you dine on garlic
you might well be a hermit.
However, not for
all the tea in china
would I allow myself
to scrumptiously indulge,
even if the proof of the
pudding was in the eating.
Anyways it would be
a pyrrhic victory.
Despite how finger
lickin' good this
damsel may be,
her dominating demeanour
was too much for my palate.
If I was to remain
worth my salt
I must suck it up buttercup
and exit quickly,
and so I did.

I was starting to
experience frustration,

perhaps even sour grapes
that I wouldn't find
my bread of life.
Life seems to be
an onion and we
cry while peeling it.
Just where is that veggie
that will make us laugh?
I was fatigued and
literally getting famished
so I sat down at the bar
and ordered spaghetti,
a meal that requires
all of my attention.
I thought of ordering antipasto
before my pasta but
questioned if that would
negate my appetite
and I'd still be hungry.
Verily, the trouble with
eating Italian food
is that five days later
you're hungry again.
I knew my worries
would go down with
a bowl of soup, so
this was my appetizer.
Pensively I recalled that
I had been taught
to practice safe eating -
always use condiments.
Perhaps for me
it was too late
to settle down.

There was no gain to
crying over spilled milk.
Anyways I continued to ponder
that man does not live
by bread alone,
when serendipitously
the toast of town
sat down by my side.

So there she was,
a natural smiling beauty,
with a long curly carrot top
framing her hazel blue eyes
offering an inviting
welcoming gaze.
Plus, no makeup.
Like butter versus margarine
I trust cows more than chemists.
She was so intoxicatingly
witty, not sarcastic,
no cheesy talk.
I knew she was
one smart cookie.
Like any smorgasbord in life
my choice was there.
In fact, it's always there,
every day, every hour,
every minute, every second.
I knew that good food
wasn't cheap,
and cheap food wasn't good.
Thus, starving for
such a companion,
and now courageously disciplined

by my fasting practice,
I chose.
Now my dinner bell of love
is hearing my name from
her lips.

True Love

We quest to find
That one of kind
From cradle to grave
The true love we crave.

But just what is that
As we sit here and chat?
Plucking daisy petals to see
She loves me not, or she loves me?

Yes love's a many splendoured thing
Inspiring poets to write songs we sing
From the very beginning and worldwide
Desiring to love and be loved as passions collide.

Some say it's the oxytocin elevation
That declares a loving mother's devotion
That mother-child bond so selfless, so strong
Perhaps only hardwired for her genes to pass on.

Then there's receptors for the hormone vasopressin
Dictating monogamy, possibly a love of repression
The dopamine reward circuit becomes stimulated
And amygdala's neuronal activity gets eliminated.

So fear is terminated and trust abounds
Negative emotions disappear and social judgment hits the clouds
Love becomes blind and physical intimacy now begins
The species is preserved and mankind in the end wins.

Such a genetic reduction and evolutionary state
Removing our choice of free will in whom we date
Men choose full lipped women, with low waist to hip ratio
Women march to broad shouldered taut bodies, and that's just so.

It's pragmatic and saves time in choosing our mate
We're attracted to dissimilar genetic complex in our date
If we keep our nasal passages clear we can sniff them out
Ovulation intensifies scents and we smell them no doubt.

The homophilic rule just doesn't apply
We'd otherwise be all gay and that's just a lie
People in gay relationships, though of the same sex
Often differ from each other in gender characteristics.

Not resembling each other is what attracts us most
Opposite skills, looks and traits, joining us coast to coast
But if we're a too well defined Mars and boundary tied Venus,

Our hopes of everlasting union will cleave love between us.

It's not our similar likes for rare steak nor rock music
Not a shared political viewpoint nor enjoying drama flicks
Not even the same sense of humour, though that certainly helps
It's how we respectfully argue, that prevents our love melts.

Sarcasm, insults and criticisms destroy
Being defensive and indignant to complaints will annoy
Passive aggressive withdrawal and not wanting to talk it out
These communicative styles aren't love songs to boast about.

Never truly saying "sorry", nor apologizing first
Interrupting, 'tit for tat' sidetracking, cause conversations to burst
Bringing up the past or threats of separation are killers
Yet repair attempts, more so accepting them, are loving builders.

Being interested to know your partner and listening to them
Affirming compliments boosts your romantic sexiness to them
Giving a helping hand, yet maybe tired and unskilled too

And there is no substitute for kindness to sing our love true.

The antonym of love for some is hate
While selfishness is amor's opposite other's will state
Perhaps being afraid of never being in love is our fate
It's really fear that is love's adversary for mates.

There's no gift higher than love the Corinthians learned
It's kind and patient, without envy, a true virtue to be yearned
Love isn't arrogant said Paul, nor seeks its interest returned
Love excuses, endures all things, never ending, never spurns.

Suspenseful thrillers, anxiety, a little dose of fear
Facilitate our lovemaking, like after an argument with our dear
However eros is one form of love say the Greeks
There is also philia, storge, xenia and - agape that we seek.

Buddhist's meditate on the ideology of loving compassion
St. John Paul II said the single reality of love has different dimensions
Without being in love our life's not fulfilled
Since God loves us all, why not seek out this thrill?

For every effect there is a cause, thus for the Big Bang too

Atheism is *Non Servium,* nor accepting that God's love made you
Genetics, hormones, believing love's hard wired chemistry-or not
Your free will to read this, is like choosing God's love-or not.

Your's

Hello my beloved, says a friend.
A friend. Who is this?
Sounds absurd.
Does a true friend exist?
What is a friend?
Such a question confirms myself, as not.
A friend loves you.
The bad are both repelled and pulled
toward His goodness.
He is dear to the good, because of His likeness.
The ill gain comfort from His careful concern.
The healthy maintain their state, through His
presence.
The ugly find their beauty through His reflection.
He appeals to the beautiful, because of His rarity.
The arrogant learn humbleness through His humility.
The condemned discover their freedom in His
mercy.
The lonely become fulfilled in the excitement of His
company.
The suspicious learn trust through His confidence
and sincerity.
Forever we can continue,
and you may well discover yourself included.

But how about He who is so multi purposed?
Does this friend begrudge this utility service?
Is a friend then, one, to whoever is in need?
In the absence of you, where goes this friend?
Does He disappear to go meet His need?
Who does He desire?
What does He need?
He does not want.
He is complete.
He is Love.
Love is God.

Original publication in 'Mentally Speaking', pp. 273, 274; by Stephen B. Stokl, M. D., Volumes

Personal

Anne

A grade eight education, but so
well learned about life.
One of eighteen, four dying
before aged four, she was
seventh of the remaining fourteen.
She was the second oldest girl,
as the eldest was sent off to be
raised by a bachelor uncle from age five.
Not uncommon in Southern Ontario for a poor
Irish Catholic family during the
Great Depression.
As to the heroine of this story,
She became the surrogate mother.
Cooking, cleaning, part-time jobs,
singing in the choir, then
in her late teens to age twenty,
made studs for army boots during WWII.
Childhood to adulthood by the time she
was nine years old.
She met the man she loved, an immigrant,
German, who flew twenty eight missions for
the RCAF in Europe.
He was hard working, mechanically skilled,
and made a dollar go a mile.

Dedicated, loyal, and faithful to her,
they remained married,
yes, happily for the majority
of their almost sixty-two years until her
death.
Before her passing, she raised four children,
all university educated resulting in careers
toward the service of others.
Raised in a Roman Catholic home herself, she truly
lived out her prioritized order of life, teaching
these principles to her children, and supported
fully by her husband.
Faith, Family, Friends, Finances in that
order, for all decisions, will give you Fun
and Freedom in your Future.
She believed that if you discipline attitude
in childhood,
you won't have to discipline behaviour
in adolescence.
Never attended Finishing School nor
read Miss Abigail's advice,
but she practiced well-bred manners,
and instilled in us those social etiquette
skills, to make us better gals and guys.
She believed she was a parent for life,
and having raised six other brothers and
sisters, she understood boundaries and how to
secure harmony with in-laws,
especially daughter in-laws.
Issues of disagreement were only
when another trespassed her legal, ethical, or
moral
values.
Then she would draw her Alamo line in the sand.

Otherwise she didn't sweat the small stuff.
Her children learned an additional principle,
sometimes the hard way,
that people will perform better, not
based on what you expect, but what you inspect.
And yes, she did inspect.
So amongst a home life of love,
laughter, music, singing, dancing,
chores and homework,
her kids, and grand kids remember
Mom's 'attitudinal' and accountability
sayings, such as;

"Use a little elbow grease."

"I've got a bone to pick with you."

"You little ham 'n egger you."

"I don't care who started it, you're both going to get it."

"Go back upstairs, find your smile,
put it on your face and then come down."

"So, what did you dream about?"

"You have to learn to play the hand you're dealt."

"Patience is a virtue, seldom found in women,
and never found in men."

"Good things come in small packages. Then again, so does poison."

"Good things come in threes."

"Bad things come in threes."

"You can't get rats from mice."

"Where there's a will there's a way."

"Anticipation is the better part of participation."

"You kids are street angels and house devils."

"C'mon there lazy bones, get at it. Don't go putting off to
tomorrow that which you can do today."

"Never go to bed angry at each other."

"Don't toot your own horn."

"Offer it up." (wanting to complain from pain after bruising yourself or skinning your knee or not being invited to the party or being assigned more work than your peers, etc.)

"There's always room for one more." (at the table)

"Stop your pouting."

"Look at your face."

"Fix your face or I'll fix it for you."

"Top of the morning to you..., and

the rest of the day to yourself." (March 17th, St. Patrick's Day)

"Holy Hannah"

"Don't get too big for your britches."

"Watch yourself or you're going to go arse over tea kettle." (if you are tripping and almost fall)

"What happened, did you fall in?" (if you're taking too much time in the bathroom)

"Just know that your clothes, your coin collections, your car, your house, that it's all just stuff. It's people that really count."

"You've made your bed, now you have to lie in it."

"May the road rise to meet you, and may you be in heaven before the devil knows you're dead."

"Oh darn..., Oh shoot..., Oh shite..., Oh fudge..., Oh my gosh."

"Be home by 11:10... NO LATER!"

"That's the pot calling the kettle black."

"Did you go tinkle?" (before a car ride)

"What's mine is mine and what's 'urine' is mine."

"Look at me when I'm talking to you."

"Shove that in your updyke."

"Cold hands, warm heart."

"What did you do, drop the stone out of your ring?" (if you're out of Mom's sight but you've dropped an object that
makes a very loud noise)

"Remember to always ask the wallflower to dance."

"You better buster or your name's Mud."

"A little bird told me something...,"

"Stop looking in the mirror."

"Babies are angels from heaven that we rent from God."

"Can't the cat look at the queen?"

"If you can't say anything good about somebody, don't say anything at all."

"As long as you're living under this roof, you're getting up and going to Mass."

"You go apologize right now and mean it."

"The greatest gift that I can give to you kids, is my Faith."

"Your Dad is very upset, he's had a terrible day at the shop...,
now go upstairs and show him your math homework."

"Don't forget to stop and smell the roses."

"Never give all of yourself, totally, to anyone. Always keep
that small part of you, for you only, that is, you and God.
It will be the spark that will ignite you
and get you over any tragedy."

She wasn't a psychiatrist, not a professor,
nor a priest.
She wasn't wealthy, not a model, but
she was a servant leader who prayed for peace.
She knew right from wrong.
Taught it, and lived it,
as best as she was able.
I knew I'd won the lucky ovum lottery.
She was my Mom.

A Personified Asymptote

You are a true bellibone
living on top of the hill
I dwell in the valley
A Micawber who loves you still

Hoping everyday I'd see you
every moment with you exhilarating
your musical laugh, intoxicating smile
my heart's desire for you bursting

Alas I'm a personified asymptote
almost there but never touching
yet love seeks the good of another
love is never self-seeking

So skipping along as I ponder
fantasizing of a possible rendezvous
imagination is such a beautiful cognition
wishing I'm part of your dream come true

A Wick From Keswick

Along the shores of Lake Simcoe
Where storms and gales erupt their blow
Windsurf, kite glide, boat cruise - your pick
Is a town with a reputation - called Keswick

A drive - thru variety store, 'Pinky's' by name
Lucky's, Krates Marina, and the five corners fame
Not just greasy spoons aligned in a row
There's sushi, plus the Corner House that attracts De Niro

Stephen Leacock, McGill's Economy Prof
Inspired a centre for the cultural lot
Lumber plaid dinner jackets and snap-on tops
Mix with Harley's bad boys and plenty of cops.

Have a donut and sip on your warm caffeine brew
The town has Coffee Time, Country Style and two Timmies too
Canadian Tire and Home Hardware are a fundamental must
And now Wal-Mart has earned the population's trust.

Winter means hockey, fish huts, sleds, and ATVs
Summer exposes skin with tattoos and bikinis
Autumn is gorgeous, a deciduous colourful delight
Spring delivers parties, mania, and fellows who fight.

Yet Larry Pastorus, So Down Low, and Bubble sing out
Such joyful music removes all Wick's pout
Roche's Point reside in their silent wealth
This down to earth town reveals our Canadian health.

Gotta Feed My Belly

Three times per day the rumblings cry out
"I've gotta a dream", I'm talking about
Forget the work, the play, the study
"Kill that hunger, gotta feed my belly."

Sex is great followed by sleep
Fun slides and rides that really go steep
Puccini and Mozart, and Barber too
Deliver musical pleasure that spring life anew.

Dostoyevsky, and Hesse, and Jerzy K.
They're all our delight, what more can we say?
Yet our alimentary canal self-preserves
The way to a man's heart calming his nerves.

Prime rib, Rack of lamb and New York strip
Make'em medium rare for a juicy trip,
Caramelize the onions and sautée the s'rooms
The saliva's running', wakens the dead from their tombs.

Penne arrabiatta accompanied by Amarone
Veal Parmigiana and Calamari à la Rome
Mista or Caesar, and Balsamic with flare

Just end with some Port and Tartufo with care.

Unagi, Roe, and Shashimi aplenty
Washed down with Sake and sake and sake,
Competes with Aloo gobi, Goat curry and Samosas
Beriani and Naan and Veggie pechoras.

Sweet and sour and bitterly nice
Quiet mastication explodes their spice
Olfactory, gustatory, even somasthetic en route
The chorus of eructation, signals diner's approve.

Published in *The Literature Gourmet Revisited*, A Canadian Anthology of Poetry and Recipes - edited and compiled by Honey Novick, pg. 83, January 2017

Ironic Age

I have a stronger tongue today
perpetually cleaning out those tiny morsels
of food
from crevices between my teeth
created by lost enamel.
Age does that.
Essentially I'm a better lover today
with such a tireless muscle that
can stroke, lick, probe,
and penetrate farther
even right to the very tip.
Like wisdom though, it rarely
attracts the smooth beautiful flesh of
a third or fourth decade year old woman.
For my integumentary organ
beguiles them not.
Such irony.

Lying Supine Is So Divine

Travelling the world and seeing the sights
London, Rome, tasting Turkish delights
Monte Carlo, Macao, the French Riviera
A camel caravan in the hot Sierra.

They all sound great, full of wonder too
Yet none compare to the beauty of you
Your smile, laughter and smooth soft touch
That's the destination I desire so much.

Beneath your squeeze and rhythmic rocking
Your sweaty facial moan, 's so exciting
For under you, lying supine is so divine
Feeling your pleasure, so sweet, so fine.

Madgie Nation

Who am I trying to impress?
Have I actually met her yet?
I really do take pleasure in my fantasy
Making love to that ineffable heavens angel sent

Dreaming being at her side under the stars
Five stars that is - Ritz, Regis and Royale
Not the time to be pusillanimous
Dedicated to seek and recognize my lovely 'belle'

For she is wonderfully formed
A genuine beauty to behold
Her smiling eyes and lips
Are for me alone she so told

I choose to dwell in this spirit with her
To roam this land of the fourth dimension
Maybe my depth of neediness fuels this quest
Nevertheless I've named my sweetheart Madgie Nation

Mona Lisa

Our sons will realize one day
The rare treasure you gave to them in play
No yelling but disciplining attitude for sure
Developing behavior and moral hearts so pure.

Welcome back Lisa, brave Lisa, Lisa
May we travel together, to Rome, Tuscany and Pisa
Though miles may separate you from me
My mind speaks poetry inspired by thee.

Amazing how I miss your smile
Your soothing voice soothes my trials
I hear you laugh as you walk and wander
Truly distance makes the heart grow fonder.

Where are you now in this world of ours?
Enjoying a margarita or shopping for hours
Sunning on the beach or visiting a ruin
Wherever you are I dream you return soon.

Nulli Secundus

No 'Bash', 'Boom', 'Kapow' or 'Zap'
This game's for real, K. O. or tap
Endurance, strength, focus, and think smart
Six inches between the ears set the champions apart
Mix muay thai, karate, wrestling, and judo
Add kick-boxing, sambo, jiu-jitsu and capoeira.

Rome's coliseum waged the gladiators of old
Now the octagon births new warriors bold
No death but violent, blood and gore allowed
Entertains armchair voyeurs filling the crowds
A young adult's game, and women too can fight
Enter with their theme song, to the audience's delight.

Why fight another person, hurt and make them bleed?
Working out a resolve, childhood conflict gives need.
Puts food on the table, a roof over your head
Increases the chance to take that one to bed.
Plus, the self-esteem spice of recognition
Rewarded to those in optimal condition.

The legendary names like Achilles and Alexander
Now are Jones, GSP, Machida, and Edgar
No trident thrust, sword, spear, or roar of tiger,
Just arm bar, guillotine, heel hook and kamikaze calf crusher.
Refereed to fair play, no biting, genitals off limit,
Not fixed, nor thrown, just Olympian credit.

Soccer takes stamina, football demands guts
Hockey is speedy, golf's won on putts.
Basketball, horseracing, excel at a height
Baseball requires coordination, chess must be right
True, tennis is man versus one on one
But the MMA champion combines all - *second to none.*

Tapp'n

Competition number five
Making those feet come alive
And if that dance goes off the track
We improv moves, to bring us back.

Bojangles, Astaire, Kelly and Hines
Mixed pas de bourée, and chaînés, together so fine
Triple pirouette, grand jeté, and aerial
So cool to create, groov'n to the stereo.

Costume change, rehearse, and edit
Signing our style, and building us credit
Tapping the beat, avoiding any feathers
Glue on the smile, aware of the others.

Pounding the boards, our feet are the drums
Spinning and jostling and twisting our bums
Its fun and alive, to speak so unique
Tap danc'n's our music, our expression so sweet.

TGIF

We partied with Black Tower, Baby Duck, and Blue Nun
Danced with Donini and Mateus til they're done
Laughing and joking over stories we told
Recalling memories forgotten of our actions so bold.

Lubricated fine, now off to make the scene
Crav'n stimulation, final make-up and preen
Got to line-up at our favourite dance club
Passport of green backs is our entry stub.

Four eyes connect across the glistening floor
She likes - he likes, what are we wait'n for?
No thoughts of studies or work'n real late
Brut meets Charlie in this heady date.

Hitting the floor and cranked up to jive
Embracing our partner, intensively alive
Red cheeks, sweaty necks, clothes getting wet
Stepping out our freedom tête à tête.

A squeeze here, a nuzzle there
Pressing our contact without a care

Hoping to remove unnecessary attire
Panting our lust with moves of desire.

The band's rock'n higher, hitting the clouds
Rav'n and gyrat'n, mass frottage in the crowd
Strobe lights, disco ball and dry ice smok'n
Saw dust, feet slid'n as we're glid'n and strok'n.

Two-thirty A.M. as we close the place down
Still smil'n and energized as we cruise around town
Don't want this TGIF night to end
Our hearts playing good times as our souls ascend.

Relationships

Alliteration Addiction

The annual award for Eve's eloquent elocution
As proudly promoted by the International Institution
Was richly rewarded to this newbie narrator
She'd captured the controlling judge's fond favour.

For she spoke on the subject of love lost and loneliness
A telling tale of humble happiness
Though robustly regaling her own personal past
This lady's lament focused ears forward and fast.

A country courtship started one sizzling summer
Powerful passion portrayed their tingling thunder
Running round and round, holding hand in hand
Broadcasting 'bella' in laughter's land.

A Mendelhson marriage mated the perfect pair
Perpetually playing with capricious care
Twosome togetherness singing side by side
'Til insidious incidents drove a damning divide.

No more cuddling comfort and thinking of thou
Covert communication and no truth to tell

Now silent and suspicious, always agonizingly alone
Her actions and antics beat him bare to the bone.

He suffered and sacrificed and endlessly endured
No medicinal mix managed to calm or cure
She cared less and little for his hurting heart
Her infidelity and indifference assaulted them apart.

Plenty of partners had penetrated Eve's pleasures
She yearned for her youth and those titillating treasures
Her personal priorities prevented a perfect past
Despite daring dream dates with a celebrity cast.

Eventually Eve recalled his honest humility
She reluctantly remained as she feared turning fifty
But he loved his lady despite her callous comments
Forever forgiving her pride and petulance.

Gravitational Relationship Laws

Am I hypersensitive, too easily offended,
hence prone to quick sadness which
instantly, and temperamentally,
is transformed into anger?
Got up early, bag packed, then
went to reconcile the hotel bill before departure.
Bought and brought back two coffee for us too.
She statingly asked,
"Can you put my laundry in your bag?"
Not even a thank you.
Immediately I was hurt and felt irate.
She had the largest luggage bag.
I purchased nothing on this trip
compared to the fall wardrobe she'd secured.
I had shortened my sleep to be prepared, set to go
so I might leisurely relax until that time.
I liked being organized and being punctual.
It's the politeness of King's.
Most knifing though was the entitled request.
No introduction of apology
despite her knowing my style,
and that I had been already ready.
No verbal inclusion to even offer an
opportunity to be heroic, to raise my
belief in my benevolence, to solidify

my self-esteem.
A simple, "Oh Hon, thanks for the coffee, I'm sorry,
you're so good, you've already packed,
is there any way you can possibly
find room in your bag for my laundry,
I'm really stuck here, but it's okay if you
can't?"
So much more tender, polite, complimentary,
creating a springboard for me to experience
some magnanimity.
I mean, that's what I would've said,
and acted, if it were me.
So what?
She's not me.
Still, after all the many things
I've done for her,
I mean surely, she could
at least speak nicely to me
just this once.
Says who?
Instead, I perceive being used,
taken advantaged and for granted.
Innumerable examples of this same discourse to count.
Yet, here I was a marital therapist.
Now what?
Do I practice what I preach?
What do I say?
Retaliate with a verbal riposte or passata sotto?
No.
Many a wise man has a chewed up tongue.
What do I do?
Pout?
Give the silent treatment?

Isolate?
Bang some table or wall?
How do I go from being hurt, accelerated
to anger, then light speed ahead to longsuffering,
forbearance, forgiveness and "offer it up", such
that my answer is, "… Sure, no problem, I'm sure
it will fit," matched by a genuine smile and
upbeat action to achieve just that.
Expectations are premeditated resentments.
I was getting my knickers in
a twist, forgetting some
basic gravitational laws of
relationship life.
You know what I mean.
The basics.
Like what goes up must come down.
No need to understand calculus,
nor Newton's formula for this force.
We can want, wish, even hope
that when the apple drops, it
falls up, but it won't.
So best to know the rules of
the game for optimal fun and play.
I needed to remember and acknowledge that
she is my spouse and not my child.
Therefore she is not looking to me for
any teaching accountability, nor guru advise
regardless of my expertise and reputation.
So too, despite my belief in my
interpersonal and conflict resolution skills,
I must also embrace that final filter,
that gravitational law of communication
between husband and wife;
if you are confident that the results of

what you are about to say, or not say,
and how you are going to deliver either,
will increase harmony between you,
rather than lower it, then proceed.
Furthermore, if in doubt, don't.
Accepting these gravitational laws of
matrimonial dynamics,
isn't an easy swallow for a weak character.
Then again this sacrament of marriage is not
for weaklings.
No trespassers please.
At least not for those who believe
that a covenant oath,
is forever.
Still knowing doesn't guarantee doing and
partners are bound to falter and at times fail.
Seventy-seven turns of the cheek, and
perpetually owning one's responsibility and
thus apologizing, eventually transforms
even the weak to become meekly strong.
As this is what we're called upon to do.
The *bonum universal*.
Not possible through our own human endeavor
and merit, but by prayer, self-restraint, and
self-sacrificial repentance, we are gifted,
divine grace to overcome
wrongful human conduct,
caused by natural human feelings.
So like Ripley you can believe this or not.
However for optimal marital love and longevity,
I'd recommend instead Thomas,
who though skeptical,
practiced, prayed and followed,
and thus heavenly became,
all yours.

Growing Older and Up

When you were eighteen, did you really think,
While puff'n a herb and sling'n a drink,
That you'd be here right now, at the point you are
Your dreams and reality split apart so far.

Hopscotch, double-dutch, pajama parties a plenty.
Then kilts, 45's, dances and feeling ready.
Chestnut Kingers, British Bulldog, yellow pee-wees kept you busy.
While hockey, playing pool, and Bond flix chilled your willy.

So college is past and you got your degree.
Got married too, now two kids to feed.
You're working your way up in that career you chose.
Focused on something, but not smelling the rose.

Writing notes to each other, texts soon to come.
Home late from work, eating supper for one.
Play briefly with kids, but blind to their cry.
The young ones grow up believing their name's "Bye-Bye".

Now money is tight and debt has dug deep.
The school called again and your pagers gone beep.
Fatigued you watch movies, but asleep by ten.
We don't talk anyways and barely seem friends.

Gained thirty odd pounds and not looking hot.
Your fantasy lover becomes a website spot.
Alcohol, gambling, and over-working too.
You've spun out of control, lost in life's zoo.

Now the prostate stalls your urine flow.
Ever since menopause her insomnia grows.
Headaches, stiffness, and even spices now hurt.
Pills of all colours remove your flirt.

Yet something's changed besides the hair growing thin.
Aware of life's preciousness and the consequence of sin.
Respect and kindness vibrates between our hearts.
And love trumps sex, as it did at the start.

We look after each other and play music again.
Grandkids come along and we dance with our kin.
Such a treat to sing ciao, ola, and hello.
Eating merriment together has nourished our soul.

Wrinkled and worn, blurred vision, our gaits slow.
It's been tragically magic with so little we know.
Yet wherever we go there we are at last.
Forgiveness is giving up hope for a better past.

I Should've Known Better

Gave me a kiss, said we'd meet at eight
Showed up at eleven, said sorry I'm late
Slept together, but left before he ate
Texted me a week later to ask for a date.

He always had a reason to leave
A card shark with an ace up his sleeve
Sweet words he'd say that I believed
Dreams of our future I would conceive.

Followed him one Saturday night as a lark
Said he was at poker with his buddy Mark
Found him with Sarah in the park
Half naked together romping in the dark.

Came dressed as a rose but was a thorn
Hello's, goodbye's and this loss I mourn
Wounded my trust and my heart was torn
Emotional scars tattooing my heart scorned.

Need to move on now, at all cost
Had cried for what's hoped for, but not really lost
Must reflect on myself for being so tossed,
Improving my lens for future love's sauce.

It's All In A Name

Frank talks were my
father's style, combined with sage
advice from my mother
Prudence.
I thought my dad was outdated,
older than Methuselah,
but I knew
he was no Nimrod.
In fact he was known
amongst his friends
as a Danny boy,
and heralded as a Lancelot
when stating his counter cultural
and politically incorrect opinions.
Still, against Justus's counsel
my dad's most proper name,
I lived my prodigal life.
I had given Rose my
everything, or so I believed.
She had known my emotional handicap,
as I had trusted her.
Yet like all stigmatizing,
she had judged, even misinterpreted
my symptoms and signs

as weaknesses of my will or character.
Just not true.
In return I had received a
'Dear John' text as this
Delilah told me she had
met another.
Scott free is perhaps
how I should have felt.
However it was a Goliath
of heart felt pain,
like a stabbing by Brutus
to my friendship.
I perceived myself as
a modern day Dick.
I isolated myself, cried,
and like Narcissus I began
to lose my will to live,
besides going through a Randy withdrawal,
I romantically despaired that I'd ever meet
my Juliet.
Fortuitously I was encouraged
by the girls with the same face
who lived next door.
They were identical twins,
Faith and Hope.
I started to believe
again in myself.
They said not all
women are a Jezebel,
nor are all men a Judas.
Love conquers inertia.
You need to just open the door a little,
as there is a whole new
world waiting for you.

They were right.
I had been struck
a self-esteem blow.
Rejection had become my
Achilles heel.
And as time passed, buoyed
by the twins' transfer
of belief in me,
I met a virtuous beauty,
Grace was her name.
and I became renamed - Victor.
And Bob's your uncle.

Joyful Travailing

Wanna make some money for my honey
Keep her skipp'n, happy, and smil'n sunny
Do whatever it takes for my cute cupcake
Cause she's my beauty, my sexy sweet cakes.

Brick lay'n, deck clean'n, pick'n up trash
Pizza deliver'n, even market survey'n for clean cold cash
Pack'n myself a wad by any legal and moral means
Just juggl'n jobs to keep the jingle in my jeans.

Buy her a rocky road in a tasty sugar cone
Or the latest purple jacket designer iPhone
A large emerald cut carat shining so bright
Fly her to exotica, or wherever 's her delight.

So off to work I whistling go
A labour of love, that only I know
Passion's will sure does always find a way
Excited by memories of our play in the hay.

Know Where You're Going

Older than she was he
Generations apart said society
Born when he turned twenty three
Now she's twenty eight but no vision to see.

Started out innocently enough
Listened to her when things were rough
Always smiled at her, and was never tough
Unlike her Dad, he had the right stuff.

Left for a drink after work one night
Made her laugh and feel so right
She felt so relaxed and not uptight
Hook, line and sinker, she did bite.

His lovemaking was both aggressive and kind
His energy and stamina were on endless rewind
He was playful on top, bottom, front and behind
She reached orgasm first and he never did mind.

The dating continued and she moved into his place
Travelled the world and lived a celebrity pace
But his children showed her an unfriendly face
His associates were nice but she felt out in space.

He started to avoid the company of her friends
He didn't like their music, seemed inflexible, wouldn't bend
Years later she'd no financial worries to fend
But the passion was gone, excuses she couldn't mend.

Now she's forty three, wiser, and a beauty still
He's sixty six, walks slowly and takes ten pills
She doesn't need him, nor his money, nor his will
She laments her choice, and the trapped boredom that kills.

Made In The Shade

I'm a blessed man.
I know I'm wanted, well
correction, needed.
I pay the hydro, gas, phone, internet,
cable, taxes, mortgage,
groceries, tuitions, books, computers,
house repairs, renos, 'creep'renos, appliances,
car insurance, gas, maintenance,
look after blue and green bins, garbage,
restaurants, ordering in, vacations,
spa cleaning, boat wear and tear
and launch and storage, Visa,
MC, AMEX and surprise mail from
HBC and Sears, switch off,
lights in rooms vacant of people,
and..., too pooped to continue.

It's good to be needed.

In return, smiles, clean clothes, tidyish house,
control of the remote
until I pass out at ten thirty, and...,
she hasn't left.
We take turns individually
sharing activities too.

Cooking, cleaning dishes and
kitchen, and...,
that's pretty good.

I guess it all equals out.

At least they complete some top
needed priorities for each of us.
I'm not counting.
I learned that if you help
someone in trouble, or in need,
they will remember you
when they're in trouble or in need
again.
Sounds cynical.
Maybe.
Its true though.

Anyways, I'll read some
good books, golf or go fishing
alone, or with a guy friend
once a week.
I've got it made in the shade.
As for love, hugs, sincere
complements and recognition,
..., well, children and work
fill these precious rocket fuel tanks.
Sex?
Well, "Hey", I say to self,
"Come on Luke, nothing is free.
You can't have such a blessed life
without sacrificing something".

So there I go.

Marital Manners

Prepared for our marriage
not our wedding day.
By compromising our 'I',
'We' will thrive and play.

A chewed up tongue
prevents our union being hung.
So let it go, just let it go
Let it go, just let it go.

Being young and beautiful,
skin turgor taut and glistening,
yet sex is only five percent of togetherness,
the top five percent for those listening.

Again a chewed up tongue
prevents our union being hung.
So, let it go, just let it go
Let it go, just let it go.

Develop a rhinoceros hide and
duck feathered back and shoulders.
Recognize sticks and stones break bones
but critical words are crushing boulders.

Yes, a chewed up tongue
prevents our union being hung.
So, let it go, just let it go.
Let it go, just let it go.

Every marital day in your first and last year
think, "What can I do to please you?'
The goal is to deliver harmony and truth.
Achieved by sustaining this final filter in all we do.

And a chewed up tongue
prevents our union being hung.
So, let it go, just let it go
Let it go, just let it go.

Remember you're different, not the same
Fanaticism starts where your interest stops.
Private time and space is needed by each.
Respecting your sports, and you her shops.

So a chewed up tongue
prevents our union being hung.
Yes, just let it go, let it go.
Let it go, just let it go.

Be a fiscal steward, and
let the most skilled manage the cash.
Materialism starts where your income ends,
thus live within your means to avoid a crash.

A chewed up tongue
prevents our union being hung.
So, let it go, just let it go
Let it go, just let it go.

Soft paws depend upon what you rub
so hold hands alot and sing together.
Going for walks, having fun surprises for your mate
secures your navigation through inclement
weather.

Thus lest I forget, a chewed up tongue
prevents our union being hung.
So, let it go, just let it go.
Let it go, just let it go.

No Malice Intended

She smiled at me and so lifted my heart
Believed she smiled only at me from the start
She laughed and giggled at my humorous way
That eighth of July was my very best day.

Waited six months before our first date
Loving someone at your work is a damn mistake
She made liver and onions which I never liked
But I gobbled up seconds to her delight.

Made love on the floor before dessert
Three more times before morning stirred
So it continued and we married next June
Yet living with her would be my ruin.

Our first born brought love like I never had
We bought a bigger house because she seemed sad
Our second girl came and we both were glad
Yet a gap had grown and I was start'n to feel bad.

Not all women desire a mother to be
Had to make her feel that her life was still free
I worked all day, cooked and changed diapers all night

Didn't mind at all, cause my three gals were doing alright.

Then came our third, our baby boy
She seemed happy again so full of joy
I got working harder the more to provide
Every spare moment I spent at their side.

Seven years later she gave me the news
"I'm not in love with you" and that's speaking true
She couldn't say where, when or why
But just being with me made her life die.

I cried, I cursed, and I felt betrayed
Neither argument nor gifts influenced her to stay
I still loved her, craved her, both body and soul
But it didn't matter, for the bell had tolled.

We split the assets and I was stabbed once more
I'm now with my kids around her scheduled tour
My heart still hurt from being so wronged
Took four more years 'til I believed I did no wrong.

However, even that rational wasn't true
We each had our agenda, her's made me blue
For people unite, stay, and separate
According to changing priorities, starting with the first date.

So keep on assessing your choice of mate
Even after that exciting first date
Gifts, acts of service, quality time and talk
Affirming words, sex, even touching while you walk.

Cause we're a mystery to ourselves let alone others
Kinda paranoid, depressed or anxiously smothered
No malice intended, no harm planned our way
We're just all a little cuckoo crazy, seeking serenity each day.

Our Agenda Doomed Our Dance

Kim was a princess, the most beautiful of them all
Her smiling face radiant, neither short nor too tall
Her tanned skin enhanced her torso's curves
Long legs meeting hips that made men swerve.

No matter what I did to win her desire
Got my Ph.D. and awards peers did admire
I worked out on weights, stayed lean and trim
Kept look'n for ways to win love from Kim.

Adorned Kim in Vuitton, Coach and Gucci
Trips to Bermuda, Rome and Bali
Tanzanite, Turquoise, Emerald and gold
T'is my sad tale, a warning to be told.

Kim never loved me but she loved to be craved
Married my security but my heart she depraved
Happy for awhile but unsatisfied, wanting more
Kim wanted novel stimulation, routine was a bore.

We looked good on the outside Kim and I
Behind closed doors she didn't even try
What to do, what to say, I felt so much shame
So I talked to no one, I was losing this game.

Kim didn't hate or love me, just tolerated my being
Though I tried with my might to be recognized and seen
She'd rather say nothing and be alone in her bed
So I accommodated to please and tears I did shed.

Indifference feels worse than not being liked
My self-esteem waned as did my belief in my psyche
Kim had what she wants not, says she's trapped in a jail
Blames me for no freedom and forever I post bail.

Kim married for richer, for health and delights
I married dear Kim for respect in her sight
Seems we both took a vow, though different you see
Our agenda doomed out dance, as together we're not free.

Quid Pro Quo

Something for something
That's *quid pro quo*
Something for something
That's *quid pro quo*

You hold her door open
To receive her smiling token

You take her out for dinner
Expecting sex that she'll deliver

Something for something
That's *quid pro quo*
Something for something
That's *quid pro quo*

Women want to dress their men
Men like to undress their women

You gladly watch that chick flick
Anything to get your dick licked

Something for something
That's *quid pro quo*

Something for something
That's *quid pro quo*

A little barter, a little trade
A little switch, a little exchange
No one gives what they don't have
I scratch your back and you scratch mine
There is no free lunch
There are always strings attached
Some are ropes, others chains
Most are invisible
No one's to blame

Something for something
That's *quid pro quo*
Something for something
That's *quid pro quo*

Purple

Roy Gbiv was how I remembered.
It had the lowest angstrom
but highest energy for sure.
Difficult dye for any man to make, and
even Jimi sang about its synesthetic haze.
Born in the amethyst month one winter
A periwinkle blanket wrapped her, and
trimmed with a mauve silk collar at the neck.
Fuchsia stockings became her favourite.
I met her when spring lilacs blossomed.
Adorned in a magenta light blouse.
We danced, drank wine and sang.
Popping grapes in each other's mouths.
Years went by without seeing her, and
I kept her lavender scarf nearby.
I agonized and suffered from her absence.
Remembering her perse gloved wave 'goodbye'.
For she was royalty, a regal beauty.
And no violet guy was I.
I did give her a ring of friendship.
Made of tanzanite, shaped in a tear.

That First Best Kiss

That first best kiss I'll never forget
Had desire for me more than my pet
A life time of seconds though we'd only just met
Then smiling as we part, my world now set.

Kiss of desire that made me swoon
Kiss of desire under a bright moon
Kiss of desire I miss so much
Kiss of desire as our moist lips touch.

That first best kiss was an entry key
That first best kiss buckled my knees
That first best kiss no one else sees
That first best kiss "...could I have more please?"

Cory was healthy and Ronnie was bright
Alex was wealthy and Sam was tight
Ashley was toned and Taylor was supple
Lauren would moan yet Bobbie did couple.

They all were fun and I learned a lot
Wild good times and never got caught
Experience and time were the teachers who taught
That first best kiss was the taste I sought.

So tell me truly in this big tiny place
How many you've forgotten as you danced and chased
Yet there's one stands out more than the rest
It's that first best kiss that beats all the rest.

There Is Only Do

You gave me your word
said you'd be true to me.
Promised your love
now and to eternity.

I kept my vow
was faithful to thee.
You said you tried
but gave your lust, not loyalty.

I wanted to believe
held hope in my breast.
You gave what you could
just failed true love's test.

Hurt me to see
you betray me with a kiss.
My gut felt so empty
fell into a deep abyss.

Promises were made
with good intent I know.
But like an arrow released
cannot return to its bow.

For few there are
whose worth is their word.
Not breaking their covenant
when their flesh is so lured.

There is no try
there is only do.
With no heart in your try
there's no tri "umph" for you.

I have learned that well done
is better than well said.
That the choices we make
directly lead to our bed.

Better to have loved and lost
than really never loved at all.
Those whose word is their worth.
their soul's integrity stands tall.

There Is Nothing Quite Like It

Her eyes met mine through the crowded maze
I hold my gaze with hope ablaze
Noise and chatter seemed to fade away
Her desire is all that matters this day

I see then the faintest sign
She doesn't drop her eyes in kind
The muscles around her lips contract
An olive branch and her smile reacts

We close the distance in no time flat
Like magnetic opposites force the attract
A foot apart now narrowing the gap
She blinks, still smiles, I'm helplessly trapped

A surge of lightning fires my veins
Her hand touches mine, extinguishing pain
So warm and soft and tender she holds
I gasp as our fingers entwine and enfold

I didn't know she felt just like me
Craving each other like the wind and the sea
Palpitations and tremors, lightheaded I felt
Passions' proximity removed angst from my belt

We walked together and with silence spoke
An alcove we reached, no anxiety our yoke
Inches away from that radiant face
No words did we speak in this sacred place

Lavender, jasmine, some vertigo bouquet
Green eyes, red lips so radiant were they
My knees buckling as my heart cried cheers
Heavens' doors opened to crush my fear

Our heads turned slightly, our eyes closed down
Heated desire guides our heart beat sounds
My mouth meets full, moist, indescribable delight
We melt as one in this beautiful moonlight

Our bodies now joined and we two have changed
There is nothing quite like it, this human exchange
Her tongue seeks and connects deeply with mine
The kiss, the kiss, that is so divine.

Original publication in 'The Warbler's Song', pg. 27; Polar Expressions, 2014

Today Is Yesterday

I can't remember
the last time,
I tasted your lips
returning love divine.

Driving a Porsche,
sipping Dom Perignon,
fishing Tahitian waters,
front 'n centre at a U2 show.

My stocks rise high,
family's health is good,
got a Board promotion,
and got my cabin in the woods.

So here I am feeling so empty,
surrounded by 'yes' men, yet so lonely.
I try my best, 'n give so desperately.
But my thoughts obsess on those yesterday's.

It's not her fault,
she just doesn't care.
Her love is her home,
decorating with flare.

How I'd love to be,
that slate tile she wants.
Or pressed to her side,
like those leathers she flaunts.

To be hugged and kissed,
like our dog she does squeeze.
I just don't have the fur,
for this woman to please.

Now what do I do?
What's the wise next move?
If it's love and not anger,
that influences my groove.

For her smile teases me,
and her laughter I adore.
She cooks my favourite dish.
Just physically loves me no more.

Well, I stick and stay, not desperately.
I get her that yacht, called, "Not Lonely".
Because hope burns eternal, not empty.
Faith wins, so fear not, today is yesterday.

Veni, Vidi, Vici

Wonderland has it's games and slides
Lots of thrills and chills to ride
Like the adventure of making a change in our life
Brings us angst and bittersweet fright.

New streets and sounds and a cool way to stride
Networking to reach society's stage of pride
As artists philosophize and hang at cafés
Rejecting the unprepared at soirées.

Taking orders from rude impatient peers
Cleaning, serving chow, and counting their beers
Striving to achieve through my relentless labour
Only broken focus will cause my failure.

Thinking strong and clear until she walked in
Blonde hair, blue eyes, curvaceous yet thin
A smiling voice that melted me away
Her words sang freely as she began to pay.

Nothing ventured, nothing gained
Believe in yourself, let muscles strain
You don't have to be great, you just have to start
Courage separates men from mice apart.

"My treat" I said "if you'll let me please?"
"Okay, but nothing comes free or with ease."
I needed a comeback, couldn't blow this chance
"How about a drink some time, or just join me in my trance?"

So off we went for an hour or three
Paradise, I didn't want it to end you see
Playful, laughing, almost skipping as we went
An angel from heaven I believed been sent.

Fame, fortune and success were my goals
No longer important, now all left on shoals
Despite plans and work I'd set and signed
My only desire was her lips to join mine.

To make God laugh, tell him your plans
Life happens as we go marching through sand
Once I only wanted material success
Now love's kiss changed me I confess.

Did I lose, or flounder or wander in jeopardy
Not at all, I found her, a miracle given to me
I set out, then saw, to conquer was for me
This unknown beauty I love- *Veni, Vidi, Vici*.

You Turn The Other Cheek

Relationships can be tough
and they rarely work as planned.
A honeymoon on the beach
can wash away like sand.

Takes compromise, commitment
and forever holding hands.
Got to take turns doing sacrifice
whether you're a woman or a man.

"Why'd you buy those shoes,
you don't need another pair?"
"Put your clothes in the laundry room,
don't throw them on your chair".
"Here's a list for you to do,
because you don't remember, you don't care."
"Stop whistling and tapp'n your fingers,
it's impossible to bare."

"You don't teach the kids enough,
you always work, you're never here."
"This place is in chaos you know,
you're always upset, never of good cheer."
"You forgot the garbage again,

I can't do everything round here."
"I work hard all day long,
can't I have a couple beer?"

Best to grow a tougher hide
keep your sense of humour at all cost.
Know your ordered priorities
or you'll end up being lost.

Relationships are great
when no one is trying to be boss.
It's greater still you know
warming with heat and not your frost.

"Those shoes look awesome Babe,
they perfectly match your dress."
"Here's a nice merlot,
Hon, I'll look after that mess"
"Sweety, don't worry about that list,
they're not that important I guess."
"You've really got rhythm you know,
you keep a beat with finesse."

"You're a great loving father,
you really devote quality time."
"When you smile and giggle Hon,
you make my clock chime."
"Amazing when you tackle a chore,
everything looks so prime."
"How about we order in tonight,
although your cooking 's so sublime."

So, you take it on the chin and you turn the other cheek.

You want to snap back but the high road you do seek.
You want to retaliate but humble posture you do keep.
Cause harmony's your goal not being right like you think.

We Are All Explorers

And so we come to an end.
Nothing like a good purge
to rid yourself of waste.
A bittersweet gastronomic relationship delight.

Seems one of us is blindsided
or perhaps one willfully blind.
Sure we can change, but,
payment for past actions may never end.

We are all explorers
sailing our own Santa Maria.
We have to plan, do, check and adjust,
learning and forgiving ourselves for hitting the
shoals.

Best to not judge lest we be judged
as hurting people hurt people.
The power of example is greater
than the example of power.

My cynical self says that a job
will take care of you better than a woman.
We need to believe in everyone, count on no one,
Fear no one and respect everyone.

We don't want to develop a hardened heart.
We want to live cheery not leery.
Yielding to our passions is the lowest slavery
even as to rule over them is the only liberty.

The Big Questions

Choose Your Eternal Thrill

Neutrons and protons even quarks too
They exist with electrons, totally true
Without them all matter would disappear
They have no choice nor do they fear.

Mankind however is different you see
Chemically composed but our will is free
Knowing right from wrong by the age of eight
The choices we make determine failure or great.

Our heart's silent 'lub-dub' beats to our grave
Busying ourselves with varied stuff to be saved
Six inches between the ears the game is played
Compelling our faith to act in multiple ways.

So if we be god and ourselves be *numero uno*
If we have edged God out to our *maxima ego*
Then we are prisoners of pride who will pay the price
It's not bad luck nor a poor throw of the dice.

We chose to boast and not give credit away
We chose to lie to make others obey
We chose to show bling when other's could not
We paid for front seats using credit not bought.

We buy things we don't need, to impress people we don't like
With money we don't have, just wanting to be alike
Such pursuit of recognition in social status
Will ultimately humiliate us, our importance becomes flatus.

Praising other's appearance with no thought of ourselves
Taking back row though having earned the upper shelves
Not spurious humbleness to really win favour
Only *humilitas veritas* lyses pride with savour.

The children of pride are not any better
Falling close to the tree they don't ever scatter
Envy is present and wanting all that it sees
It's color of green opposing nature's scenes.

Not happy with her house, her in-laws is bigger
Not content with his wheels, his colleagues are faster
When a friend of our's succeeds, something in us dies
And we sure feel pleasure over our friend's demise.

Fear again dominates and guards our jealous coat
But aren't we all seasick and in the same boat?
We need to complement and admire our neighbor's traits
Spread not gossip, just swallow it quickly to develop good taste.

Anger is pride's kin that we all justify

Wrath at being assaulted, betrayed, and unjustly criticized
We want our revenge and witness our injurer's torment
Vengeful thoughts obsessing us like a tangling serpent.

Anger physically destroys the vessel it's stored in
Choking our communication with everyone from within
This cycle of violence will continue uninterrupted
If dusk settles on our anger even after we parted.

The treatment is that the injured offers mercy and forgives
Seventy-seven times, or for as long as we live
Burying the hatchet gives hope for a better past
Only loving our enemy will hurdle our impasse.

Another child of pride is mediocrity's friend sloth
Pronounced long or short, to decide is a challenging oath
This is the noon day devil, being quite bored and indifferent
Fearing controversial opinion, lacking initiative even diffident.

Not taking a side as relativism 's our way
However standing for no truth, we'll fall any day
Here for a good time, cruising, "no pressure please"
Our value equals their value said absolutely with ease.

Thus wandering in emptiness, questioning heaven sent
Remedied by purpose, a mission, since life 's not lent
Our lazy attitude is defeated by zeal for our quest
We proceed with haste, passionately performing our best.

Avarice is another spawn of our deadly pride
Possessed by our desires causing our ambitions to collide
An unreasonable need to hoard plenty of riches
Despite not filling our void, yet controlled by greedy wishes.

It's not the clinging to wealth that fear shouts we should
Justly go and build profit, but for the common good
Generously helping humanity, whilst not forgetting our neighbour
The secret of living is giving, granting us peace, making us braver.

Next in the sib line is the appetite of gluttony
Whose good reason is trumped by passion's pleasures, not satiety
Consuming food and drink and stretching our belly
Our intoxicating addiction turning mind and body to jelly.

Our thirst, our hunger are malfocused thus not fulfilling

Our temple 's not cared for, surrendered to compulsive craving
Only by disciplining harmful pleasures with restraint will we last
Self-denial produces a healthy future, won by our fast.

And last but not least is the spoiled son of lust
He uses women pretending love, but really destroys trust
He treats another person not as an end, but as a means
The objectification of another to please his fantasy's needs.

Sexual uprightness is meaningless in his diabolical deceit
Sizing up all feminine beauty like meeting meat to eat
Ignorant of true love for oneself and another
He needs to be chaste and respectful, to the otherness of others.

In marriage too she may be used as our orgasmic toy
A true man will recognize this, but certainly not a boy
So if we succumb to lust, which is not a victimless crime
Seek out SLAA groups, seek purity before it's too late, it's time.

It's a journey of learning this precious life of ours

Our suffering trials produce patience and we know not our hour
Faith determines our belief, but our will conducts what we'll do
God judges our sin and virtue, so choose your eternal thrill.

How We Will Dash

Run and stay busy to avoid the fear
Avoiding those thoughts that bring us to tears
Altogether alone we're in this time
Hoping our faith will bring truth sublime.

Don't want to think about the kids getting hurt
Don't want to think about my wife and her flirt
Don't want to think about losing my folks
Don't want to think rather hide behind jokes.

Got to be masochistic to work with the ill
Suffering and sadness unhealed by a pill
Crazy way to make money treating others' distress
Forever in business cause this world's a mess.

Gotta be more than our senses perceive
Didn't know in utero what I now believe
Thought I had figured it out before puberty began
Now sex and money dictates our life's brand.

So we die and onward we go
Where we end up, nobody knows
Depends on our creed how we will dash
Our belief influences attitude about love, sex and cash.

It's Showdown

The time will come for you to choose
Your mind cries out, "refuse to lose"
If anger, hate, despair, pave the way
Conflict and confusion cries "wrong way".

Goose bumps, butterflies, nausea are felt
The struggle increases, your resolve melts
You question your courage, your vision blurs
Fear-chilling sweat, as the grim reaper purrs.

This scene's familiar and you've been there
A gossip to join, slander to share
Tax evasion, lying, a mistress to call
All forks in the road of your life's ball.

Rationalize, justify, accountability pursues
Will makes the choice and selects the cruise
The battle's begun, it's between the ears
Any logic accepted, to bury the fear.

One more taste, one last fling
Indulging yourself is your favourite thing
One more chance, that's all you want
"I'll start tomorrow", your promise haunts.

Something's different, something's changed
It's for real, the end of the range.
Darkness is looming, I'm here, only me
Yet the light keeps burning, letting me see.

For its showdown time and alone I'm not
A truth I learned, a *veritas* taught
Confidence surges, faith beats sin
The power of right, chooses to win.

It Takes Time To Understand

You need to get your work done
And must meet those deadlines
Respond to those emails
Within minutes or real time.

Yet it's the smile of your colleague
That lubricates our effort
It's that hallway chat and small talk
That soothes work's toil bringing comfort.

It takes time to understand a person
It takes time to understand their heart
It takes time to know their interests
It takes time but it is worth the start.

Amongst a group of others all strangers are we
And I'm just a newbie as well you see
Then someone cracks a joke, subtle, witty and pure
I connect and laugh together on their wavelength's humour.

Math, music and laughter are universal languages we seek
And being schooled isn't just being educated to speak
So varied our melanin, yet we be all the same
Faith in love alone, ultimately in us will sustain.

This Deal's Okay

One good turn deserves another,
was not a philosophy taught by my mother.
Instead, a gift given is a gift gone,
and offered anonymously, unconditionally,
is the sweetest song.
Not waiting with open palms
for reward or recognition,
nor applause from all to show.
Doing the right deed, with no strings attached.
Unsung.
Your ten kind acts of service to another,
entitles you to not even
one similar return from a brother.
You can only hope for
such reciprocation, or better
still, that your example is
paid forward.
Desired, yet unconscious expectations,
are premeditated resentments.
Life delivers bad things
to good people,
and serves up good things,
to bad people.
So, we don't deserve,

anything.
We may sometimes earn,
some things.
We may sometimes be
punished, exiled, or disqualified,
unjustly.
Unearned accolades and fortunes,
undeserved cruelty and illness,
that's called living.
It's not how hard we fall,
it's how quickly and high we bounce back.
Even that ability,
is not deserved,
by any of us.
However, it can be learned.
Yes, character resilience is earned.
Now when you embrace,
that this deal 's okay, you start feeling good,
really good,
and continue your *consectatio*
of happiness.

Post Mortem Credo

There is only annihilation for us,
believes the nihilist.
The hedonist disagrees, saying
we all enter an afterlife of bliss.

Both philosophical creeds
dismiss our choice.
Our decisions, our will,
have then no meaningful voice.

Thus it just doesn't matter,
we become forgotten dust or spirits of pleasure.
We can deceive, commit murder, even suicide,
anything is allowed to secure our earthly treasure.

We just need to avoid getting caught,
so as to avoid penalty and to not suffer,
our man made laws of punishment,
for our behaviour to our brother.

Seems the more money we have,
we believe the more superior that we are.
Hence the greater our corporal comforts,
convinces our own mind that we're superstars.

We recognize many
who live this way.
Yet offering them a different
creed, there belief still stays.

It's difficult for the rich and
the powerful to change their conduct.
Hell is easily rationalized away,
just doesn't exist, they don't buy it.

Begs the question of what good God
allows such an end for those He created.
However on the contrary, if Hell didn't
exist, God 's not good, its heavenly stated.

Because in the end when we die,
what if we all go to heaven?
Our choices must then mean nothing,
nor our behaviour toward our brethren.

If we all are hard wired in the end,
to embracingly accept God's mercy, love, and beauty,
then He's removed our free will, that is
our ability to choose foolish or wisely.

Thus it'd matter not at all
our previous impulses or decisions.
For we'd all have a free entry ticket,
no matter what idol we're kiss'n.

Then why let us decide
imperfectly and subsequently suffer?
Why not override our will earlier,
to prevent us from hurting others?

Is God an evil monster, a tyrant
to allow us to live this way?
Does He only overwhelm us with His love,
in the end, just to choose Him anyway?

Is this His tyranny of love which
causes us pain through our earthly life?
For any removal of our free will through terror, or
government, or even His love, makes tyranny rife.

Is there anywhere else that our
decisions and choices don't matter?
In our dreams of course, both terrible
and pleasant, though we'd love only the latter.

However, it's only a dream you know,
it's not real, it doesn't matter.
So is our life a dream of suffering, a heinous
nightmare?
Are we robotons without free will, destined to a
somewhere?

No, we choose, yes
we freely decide, even in the end.
We follow either 'Thy will be done',
or 'I'll do it my way' as our flesh won't bend.

We, not God, in our conduct choose Hell, just
like a son who chooses not his father's
righteous way.
His father says, "Alright then, your will be done",
and sadly, but true, it happens every day.

Remote Control

Like to believe
we're in control.
Not wired nor fated
to act,
by a genetic message,
forming a hormonal, neurotransmitter
concentration combination.
Strings being pulled by another,
imprinting an encrypted code
of polymorphic snips,
yet still,
it's engineered by another,
as we puppet our life's dance.
We know that's not true.
There is no remote controller.
We are in control.
We choose.
This isn't tantamount to
there being no creative designer.
Unlike instinct
installed into beasts,
we've been anointed with
the final filtering allele,
of free will.

So 'Willy' is in the cockpit
Ask most guys.
He's got his chair.
Lazy, easy, pillowed.
Tallboys, crunchie and salty treats
at his favourite side table.
And then,
power on.
FFS as the channels
speed by.
Action, gore, sci-fi
will also do.
Vicariously involved, voyeuristically glued,
minimal analysis required.
Yet, therapeutic.
He chooses to watch,
or not.
He chooses his path
along the moral conflict highway.
Not forced, nor wired,
nor chemically induced.
His conduct is not 'nilly-Willy'.
Its 'free Willy'.

Truth

We want the truth,
so we say,
the emet,
the whole truth,
and nothing but,
no hearsay.
Yet our actions speak
not to this ideal pursuit.
We extrapolate known knowledge
as our own truth,
the forbidden fruit.
For the truth is, that we live
believing what we want to believe,
not even accepting facts
too true to conceive.
A full moon increases volume
and acuity of patient emergency visits,
especially mental illness crises,
together with chaotic staff fits.
Not true.
A positive attitude
can thwart cancer, and men
with low testosterone have no power.
Not true.

Territories with restrictive
gun control laws,
have the lowest rates of murder,
and violent crime too is paused.
Not true.
Correcting a problem in
your weekend golf swing,
is easily corrected by
doing what comes naturally.
Not true.
Instead there are other truths
always operational and present,
like gravity,
and practising their teachings,
reduces hubris,
enhancing life's possibilities.
Like, people will tend to do,
what we inspect, not expect.
That people don't remember all
you've done for them,
only the feeling they last had
when you were with them.
That those who can, do
and those who can't, teach
and those who can't do either,
criticize as they preach.
That an optimist doesn't believe
everything is good,
they instead have a pre-determined belief
that there is good in everything.
That forgiveness, all enjoy.
Yet it is a virtue we most least employ.
That yes, the truth will,
set you free.

However, know that it will hurt first,
it's the key to be.
Recognizing truth in itself
is so difficult to accept.
We waffle, justify, capitulate,
whenever necessary
for our rationale to be kept.
Truth cannot be given to you.
Yet once known, it can
never be taken, so true.
The revealed truth for some children,
is a supernatural Person.
Such insight for many rich and educated,
seems only to worsen.
However, our time's coming,
in an hour, later today,
tomorrow, perhaps next month.
Like a thief in the night.
Though we live as
though we are immortal,
last time I checked, mortality
was still one hundred percent.
None of us are getting
out of here alive.
Best be certain of
our activity, nine to five,
and for heaven's sake,
live truthfully,
in order to thrive.

What's It Going To Be

More often now,
then only now and again,
I ponder what will get me,
how I will go in the end.
Eighty 's way too young
and being just beyond fifty,
I see that sure and clear.
Yet when I was twenty, reaching
forty meant less than my next beer.
So what'll it be, a massive
stroke in the night?
How about gripping chest pain
then die from an MI after the fright?
Could be no breath from pneumonia,
still a killer today.
Or uncontrolled blood sugar
amputating feet, then legs,
going blind and next,
dialysis three times per week
to keep death at bay.
Suicide 's out,
no need to make it easier for the grim reaper.
Paying more now for organic,
and multiple meals daily,

is healthy and not plain chic.
Exercising more religiously
though my belief in God varies constantly.
So all this effort, with supplements
and meditation too,
there's still my genetic heritage,
which mixed with environment,
will turn me blue.
Grandpa lived until ninety-five and both
my parents are alive and well.
I'm worrying about my life,
yet haven't crystalized my faith in heaven and hell.
Of course how could I forget it'll
probably be the big 'C'.
Lungs, liver, brain, or bone or
being found too late,
lying deep against the spine,
in the pancreatic sea.
Fretting doesn't help,
it just brings me closer to the grave.
Perhaps living life more fully,
so I won't even notice the event,
like the honourable and the brave.
Although I can't choose when,
nor what, nor where
it is going to be,
hopefully I can choose how
I'll meet my finish, and
pray I'll be a loving influence
on my family.

Biography

Born and raised in Hamilton, Ontario, Canada, Steve Stokl is an Adjunct Assistant Professor, Faculty of Medicine, Department of Psychiatry, University of Toronto and has been the Chief of Psychiatry for the past nine years at Southlake Regional Health Centre, Newmarket, Ontario. In 2007 he authored the book, 'Mentally Speaking' which was awarded first place in the category of Body, Mind, and Spirit by ForeWord Magazine. Steve is the privileged and blessed father of Zackary (and daughter-in-law Cassandra), Travis, and Jacob, and grandfather of Tirzah and Asher. He joyfully resides with his best friend, his bride Lisa, on the southern shore of Lake Simcoe in Keswick, Ontario.

Critical Praise

Stokl turns a few words into a whole story in every poem: like Hemingway's, "For sale: baby shoes, never worn." He covers more about life than most of us would see in two lifetimes.

> - Shawn Whatley, MD
> (Author of 'No More Lethal Waits- 10 Steps to Transform Canada's Emergency Departments')

Dr. Stokl's poetry provides us with an acute awareness of the foibles and predicaments of being human. Through the lens of his patients' personalities and journeys, his writings continue to mentor and therapeutically guide others to find their truth.

> - Barbara Anschuetz
> (Clinical Director, The Trauma Centre; Sharon, ON)

A delightful work of poetry that has something for everyone: wit, nostalgia, and wisdom that could only be the fruit of many years of reflection on the meaning of suffering and human well-being.

> - Deacon Douglass McManaman
> (Author of 'The Logic of Anger' and 'Why Be Afraid')

www.ingramcontent.com/pod-product-compliance
Lightning Source LLC
LaVergne TN
LVHW041626060526
838200LV00040B/1455